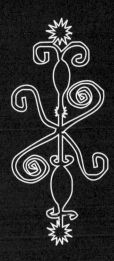

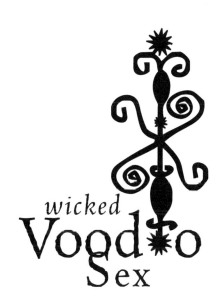

wicked
Voodoo
Sex

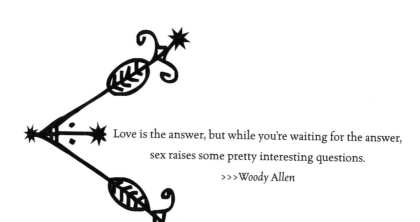

Love is the answer, but while you're waiting for the answer, sex raises some pretty interesting questions.

>>> Woody Allen

About the Author

Kathleen Charlotte is a therapist, healer, and relationship counselor who lives in England. She has practiced magic since she was a child, and she grew interested in Voodoo in the late 1990s when she visited the island of Haiti with a friend. She returned in January 2000 and initiated into its healing arts, becoming a Voodoo practitioner herself. She now combines psychology, relationship advice, and old-fashioned magic to help clients find love, keep love, and let go of love—the Voodoo way.

Kathleen is also the author of *Va-Va-Voodoo* and, with Ross Heaven—the author of *Vodou Shaman* and *Plant Spirit Shamanism*—she is a director of the Four Gates Foundation, Europe's leading organization for the teaching and promotion of spiritual wisdom and freedom psychology.

The Four Gates runs workshops in shamanism, healing, love, and relationships, as well as correspondence courses in the shamanic and magical arts. It also produces a drumming tape that you can use to accompany the shamanic and Voodoo journeys described in Kathleen and Ross's books. For more information on this and other Four Gates activities, visit www.thefourgates.com.

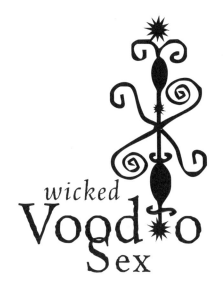

wicked
Voodoo
Sex

>>>Kathleen Charlotte

Llewellyn Publications
Woodbury, Minnesota

FIRST EDITION
First Printing, 2008

Cover design by Kevin R. Brown

Cover image of woman by Stockbyte

Illustrations by the Llewellyn Art Department

Llewellyn is a registered trademark of Llewellyn Worldwide, Ltd.

Cover model used for illustrative purposes only and may not endorse or represent the book's subject.

The material in this book is not intended as a substitute for trained medical or psychological advice. Readers are advised to consult their personal health care professionals regarding treatment. The publisher and the author assume no liability for any injuries caused to the reader that may result from the reader's use of the content contained herein, and recommend common sense when contemplating the practices described in the work.

Library of Congress Cataloging-in-Publication Data

Charlotte, Kathleen, 1960–
Wicked voodoo sex / Kathleen Charlotte.—1st ed.
    p.   cm.
Includes bibliographical references and index.
ISBN-13: 978-0-7387-1200-0
1. Sex instruction for women. 2. Voodooism. 3. Sex. I. Title.
HQ46.C39 2008
306.77—dc22
                            2007034199

Llewellyn Worldwide does not participate in, endorse, or have any authority or responsibility concerning private business transactions between our authors and the public.

All mail addressed to the author is forwarded, but the publisher cannot, unless specifically instructed by the author, give out an address or phone number.

Any Internet references contained in this work are current at publication time, but the publisher cannot guarantee that a specific location will continue to be maintained. Please refer to the publisher's website for links to authors' websites and other sources.

Llewellyn Publications
A Division of Llewellyn Worldwide, Ltd.
2143 Wooddale Drive, Dept. 978-0-7387-1200-0
Woodbury, MN 55125-2989, U.S.A.
www.llewellyn.com

Printed in the United States of America

Dedications and Thanks

For Jo, Amelia, and Ocean.
And for Camilla, Madeline, Emily, Javen,
Alex, Nathan, Mom and Dad, my sister and brother,
and all the people who've been there for me.

Contents

3. How to Kiss like a Pro (And Other Things Your Body Can Do)...57

4. Getting Your Freak On: Fantasy Favorites and Filthy Language...93

5. When I Get That Feeling, I Need Sexual Healing...119

6. Sex That's Out of This World!...157

7. Make Love, Not Laundry...183

Appendices

Disclaimer

The techniques, recipes, and approaches in this book have been tested in many real-life applications and no harm has ever arisen as a result (most people have benefited enormously). It is important, however, to act sensibly and responsibly when undertaking spiritual, sexual, or emotional discovery work of any kind. It is also important that you double-check all formulas and recipes given in this book for safety before using them internally or externally.

If you are in any doubt about any of the practices or recipes in this book, please seek medical advice to reassure yourself that there are no contraindications.

Any application of these exercises is at the reader's own risk, and the author and publisher disclaim any liability arising directly or indirectly from them, their use, or the recipes described herein.

Enjoy your Voodoo responsibly!

Foreword

This book about sex and relationships is special. It's playful and serious at the same time. It includes love spells and sex magic and information about sexual freedom from a playful perspective.

What a novel concept!

In my work as a Tantra coach, I advise people to bring back the beginner's mind. Come to the bedroom with no expectations. Come with openness in your hearts for whatever happens.

Playfulness can empower you sexually, and that is precisely what's needed. After all, there is so much baggage attached to human sexuality.

For centuries we've been taught to be against our bodies. We're piled high with shame about our bodies. And we feel guilty for wanting sensual and sexual pleasure. How can we possibly function in this type of schizophrenia? Truth be told, we cannot.

Didn't we come from sexual energy? Isn't it sexual energy that gets transformed into love? If we are against sex, how can love ever develop? We usually don't see the obvious: that we've been set up against our own energy. We've been taught "sex is sin." So we end up feeling this deep inner conflict to fight against our sex but to love at the same time.

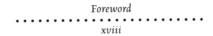
Since as humans we can never be separated from sex, since we are born out of it and it is the primary life force in all of us, shouldn't we drop the conflict? Shouldn't we focus our energy and attention on working through what has been handed to us so we can come to terms with our nature?

I say yes. I say let's look at ourselves for who we are. Let us unmask the secret that the world has been trying to hide from us. We are sexual beings, so we might as well admit it.

Rather than being obsessed with sex because we've been forced to suppress it in order to function in this world, why not have some fun with it instead? Once we know it is our true nature—the basis of all life, all creation—can we please drop the craziness, the obsessions, and just have fun? Can we drop the hatred of our beautiful bodies and learn to enjoy them with all the gusto in our hearts?

Wicked Voodoo Sex is exactly the place to start.

In my book, I state, "Intimacy with another requires, first and foremost, coming to peace with your own emotional and physical needs. This is not a small task, but it is a crucial one. It takes time and courage and forgiveness coming from you to you. If you want a sexually electric and truly intimate love affair, you have to begin unblocking and unleashing the sex force that is living inside you."

Here in *Wicked Voodoo Sex* you just may find some of the answers to unblock your vital life force, your birthright energy. You may begin to laugh and play with what is at your very core. You will find magical tools to make you more loveable to yourself and others. You will embrace your body and the lovely, juicy, sexual energy that surges throughout. What fun!

Laurie Handlers

is the author of *Sex & Happiness: The Tantric Laws of Intimacy* (Butterfly Workshops Press, 2007). Her website is www.sexandhappiness.com.

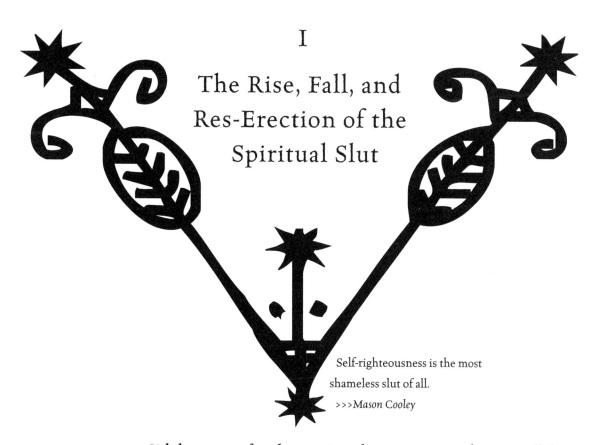

I

The Rise, Fall, and Res-Erection of the Spiritual Slut

Self-righteousness is the most shameless slut of all.
>>>*Mason Cooley*

Girls have seen a few changes since the 1960s. For one thing, we call them women these days, and they're not quite the spare ribs they once were. The twenty-first-century woman, as the great sex guru Cyndi Lauper proclaimed, wants to have fu-u-u-n—and knows (theoretically, at least) how and where to get it. But the question remains: is she really getting that much—in the bedroom, I mean? And if not, why not?

>>>

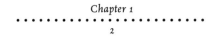
Despite all the progress women have made in matters of love and lust, men are still the dominant sex when it comes down to sex and see themselves as the ones in control because they have the testicles. Well, screw that!

My view is simple: if you've got a sex organ, it's there for a reason and you're entitled to use it. And I hope this book will help you do exactly that, by:

- Improving your sexual and magical skills through Voodoo tricks, Tantric practices, and techniques to make sex (even more) fun;

- Improving his sexual skills by showing you a few techniques you can teach him during love-making rituals;

- Helping you to stand proud and erect as a spiritual slut— and giving you some good reasons why you should;

- Initiating you into Goddess energy; and

- Turning you both on to sex as a holy, healing, and wholesome activity that is totally natural, endlessly fascinating, fabulously funny, and—amazingly—still tax-free!

In case I haven't been clear so far: women have the right to enjoy their sexuality and to experiment as much as they like in the boudoir—and it's nobody's business but theirs. There; I've said it. Women are allowed to have sex. In fact, they can even enjoy it!

If you find that a bit of a stretch—and believe me, some women still do!—look away now, because it's going to get much, much worse. Return this book to the shelf where you found it, and back away slowly. There'll be one on knitting in an aisle nearby.

Actually, no matter what women say, how coy they sometimes get, or how innocent they pretend to be about such "men's things" as sex, we all know the truth really, don't we? We like sex.

In fact, if you look back not that far in history at those old sepia photographs of pioneer families and mountain settlers—the ones who made America great in the days before the pill—every woman had a family of twelve, a baby at her breast, and a bun in the oven as well. I think it was the law in those days that Ma Walton held up her knickers with yo-yo elastic.

These recent figures from Amora, the new London Academy of Sex and Relationships, speak for themselves: women enjoy sex as much as men.

- On average, every man and woman has had ten sexual partners

- 44 percent of women have had a one-night stand

- 9 percent of women have had so many sexual partners they can't even remember the number, let alone their partners' names

- And 72 percent of women masturbate at least twice a month (which must mean, on average, that some of you are doing it on a daily or even an hourly basis)

But even with all that going on, women have never been very comfortable in admitting that they like sex, being open about their sexuality, or asking for what they want. The reason for that is social and religious pressure. If women use the S word (Sex), they're rewarded with another S word (Slut)—and so are men (Stud), who get to be quite Something by bedding them. There's still a double standard, for sure, which leads to another S word for many women: Shame.

In her book *Slut! Growing Up Female with a Bad Reputation*, Leora Tanenbaum writes that "two out of five girls nationwide have had sexual rumours spread about them. Three out of four girls have received sexual comments or looks, and one in five has had sexual messages written about her in public areas." It beats me why something as natural and wholesome as sex is regarded as a weapon of mass destruction like this, but it is.

The women Leora interviewed for her book differ in ethnic background, age, and economic status, but they all share one thing in common: each of them—along with Leora herself—was labeled a slut in school for being open about sex. "As such, they became victims of a double standard that winks at sexual promiscuity among teenage boys but insists that young women remain virginal and pure."

As Anita Hill and Monica Lewinsky demonstrate, it's not just in high school that this comes up as an issue either. Successful, professional, high-status, fully grown, independent women exercising their right to choose still get the word *slut* thrown at them if they dare to have sex and speak of it—unless you're Samantha from *Sex and the City*. But that, of course, is a work of fiction.

But let's just stop for a moment and look at this word *slut* before we allow ourselves to be shamed by it.

Thank the Goddess for Sluts

Take a look at history—and this time at herstory—and you'll find that "sluts" were once held in high regard by men and women alike. They were oracles (pythonesses) and healers who cared for the soul and brought wisdom and well-being through the power of sexual healing. Tender, enlightened, sassy, and sexy, they were regarded as the earthly embodiment of Aphrodite, the goddess of love and beauty herself. Sluts spent their days in temples as priestesses and were known as the *Horae*. Many became rich and were sought after as wives.

Some of the Horae were skilled in astrology (a profession from which we derive the word *horoscope*) and were called the Watchers of the Stars and the Keepers of Hours. Others spread love and healing as ambassadors of the goddess and were called the *Pornai*. So when you embrace your spiritual slut, you are performing a sacred act that uses sexuality as a healing and spiritual force.

In the days of the Horae, there was no virtue in virginity. The goddess of lushness, fecundity, new life, union, and growth saw no value in that. It takes the coming together of male and female (literally), after all, for things to be born and to flourish and grow. Because of this, even brides-to-be would spend seven nights at a temple under the guidance of a priestess and "sex therapist" to learn the arts of love before they married. This also appealed to the goddess—who didn't think much of marriage, by the way, because it made a woman housebound and a servant to her husband instead of the divine force itself.

Everything went along just fine like this—until Christianity. This new Johnny-come-lately religion was led by people who found the body kind of dirty (and still do, in some cases) and were more interested in mortifying their flesh than enjoying it. After that, sexual power and powerfully sexy women became the villains of history. The Horae became "whores" and the Pornai became "pornographers"—and we got a god in place of the goddess, with all of the hang-ups men usually have.

Christianity, however, is simply the retelling of much older creation myths that had been around for centuries before Christ came along—such as that of Horus, god of the sun (rather than the son of god), whose miracle birth to Meri on December 25 was announced by a bright star and who went on to have twelve disciples and change the world—all of this, incidentally, 1,000 years before Christ was said to do the same thing.

Importantly, these earlier creation stories nearly all saw women as more powerful—and inherently more sexy—than men. Another example is Lilith (who became the sanitized Eve of the Bible), who does little else all day than have sex with her hundreds of lovers because her husband, Adam, just wasn't man enough for her. Stories like these not only depict sex as A-OK, they also depict women as much more sexually free and capable than men because, for one thing, they could make babies by immaculate conception (i.e., with no need for men *and* without having to lie in the damp patch).

When you're rewriting history, however, a little demonization of women and sex (and sometimes of gay men as well) can't do any harm. And so, once

Christianity appears, we read in the Bible that "only the young girls who are virgins may live" (Numbers 31:7–18) and that "if evidence of the girl's virginity is not found, they shall bring the girl to the entrance of her father's house and there her townsmen shall stone her to death" (Deuteronomy 22:20–21). Nice.

St. Paul goes on to tell us that no good Christian should ever "suffer a woman to teach, nor to usurp the authority over a man, but to be in silence." He also has some good advice for men who get excited at the thought of sex: "I would that they were even cut off which trouble you" (1 Timothy 2:12 and Galatians 5:12)!

But perhaps St. Clement of Alexandria puts it best: "Every woman should be filled with shame by the thought that she is a woman."

Unless you're after the title of Miss Deuteronomy 2008, you might have a few problems with some of these ideas, and yet many otherwise intelligent people still live according to such "biblical truths" and have decided on shame, guilt, sexual repression, and (not-much-of-a) life everlasting instead of a healthy, natural sex life.

It was during the rise of Christianity that Hor houses (the temples of the Horae) became "whorehouses" and sex was paid for by the hour (a corruption of another sacred custom where, during the night, the Hours—priestesses who danced for the blessings of the people—would weave their sacred dance).

In fact, the words we use today to describe the once-revered profession of holy slut are all negative and hide the truth of the power of women and sex. Indeed, the one thing that women are brought up to want to be these days—

wives—was a word that in goddess culture was connected to bondage. To have a husband meant to be "housebound," i.e., tied to the *hus*, the family home where the man who owned it was god. *Marriage* meant "man's age," the age at which a woman was ready to be bound to a man.

With all the moral weight of Christianity bearing down on them, it's not surprising that women have given up sex in the last 2,000 years—or if they are having sex, it's not something they shout much about.

Help is at hand, however, because in Haiti there remains to this day a hidden society within Voodoo that exists to preserve the teachings of the Horae and their practices of sexual magic. It is called the Sisterhood of the Miracles of Night, and through its secret knowledge, you can reclaim your power and start your own sexual revolution to become the wholly happy, holy healing slut the goddess always intended you to be!

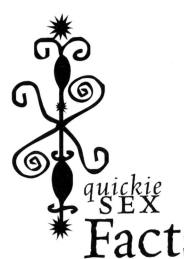

quickie **SEX** Facts!

SEX HEALS

- Kissing (and oral sex) keeps you looking younger! It exercises nearly forty different facial muscles—more than any other activity
- Men who ejaculate five times a week are 30 percent less likely to develop prostate cancer
- A magazine survey of more than 100,000 married women found that the happiest were those who could "express sexual feelings"

The Sexy Sisters of Miracles

Voodoo is the spiritual tradition I was initiated into on the island of Haiti eight years ago. I got into it almost by accident after following a lifelong interest in magic when, more or less by chance, I took a holiday with a friend in the late 1990s, and we ended up in Haiti, the home of Voodoo. It was then that I first heard rumors of a mysterious group called *Sè Mirak Lanuit*: the Sisterhood of the Miracles of Night.

My interest was piqued because back home in the UK I was working as a psychologist, relationship counselor, and sex therapist (I still do), and the practices I was hearing about that the sisterhood were supposedly experts in seemed similar to my own work but also contained a magical content I was unfamiliar with.

On that trip I was unable to learn much more about the sisterhood, but I was so impressed by the spectacle and effectiveness of Voodoo that I went on to initiate and learn its secret arts. I've found that by incorporating Voodoo techniques, spells, and practices into my relationship counseling work, the results have been pretty amazing, and I've related some of these in my book *Va-Va-Voodoo* (Llewellyn, 2007). Voodoo works! I know that from experience. But I was still intrigued by the sisterhood, and wanting to know more, I returned to Haiti again—and again: five times in all between 2001 and 2006—to see what I could discover.

Through dogged detective work, unusual coincidences, and the doors that open into a secret world when you become a Voodoo initiate, I eventually found a woman—a very wise and incredibly ancient *mambo* (Voodoo priestess) called Marie—who could lead me to the sisterhood. What I discovered was a society of female initiates who guarded their secrets and their very existence so well that even within Voodoo today they are regarded more as legend than reality.

Through my studies with the sisterhood, I learned that their practices stem from the work of the Horae in the temples of Aphrodite, going underground with the rise of Christianity and migrating to Haiti, as many other traditions did (Voodoo being a rich blend of African spirituality, European paganism, and African shamanism, among other things), and that their secret knowledge could lead to better sexual performance, more orgasms, greater personal freedom, a better time in the bedroom, and—just as importantly—to healing and spiritual growth.

I'll tell you more about the sisterhood and will be passing on their wisdom (as well as my own psychological and sex-counseling knowledge) throughout this book. First, though, I want to clear up some standard misconceptions about Voodoo, because most people hear the word and immediately get images of bloody sacrifices, mad sex orgies, and pins sticking out of dolls. Right off the bat, let me tell you Voodoo isn't like that. It's all about love.

As I wrote in *Va-Va-Voodoo*, there's no animal sacrifice in Voodoo apart from a once-in-a-blue-moon church picnic where a kindly farmer might give the congregation a ropy old cow that's no longer producing milk; then they might have a barby. But it's not done often, and no animals are simply killed as part of a blood-letting frenzy. Haiti is a third-world country and a rural community, so killing animals for food is natural, but it's never done wastefully because the people just can't afford it.

There are no mad sex orgies either (more's the pity). We are, after all, talking about a religion here, so if you wouldn't get a blue-rinsed orgy led by the priest of your local Anglican mission (which, personally, I'd love to see), there's no reason to expect one in Voodoo either.

And there are no pins in dolls. Period. It just doesn't happen in Haitian Voodoo, no matter what you've seen on the telly.

If that's disappointing, I apologize, but I'll try to make up for it later with lots of explicit sex. On the other hand, if you're still alarmed by the word Voodoo, just think of it as magic instead (because that's what it is)—or, if you're familiar with Wicca or shamanism, you'll find a lot in common with those traditions, so mentally delete the word *Voodoo* and substitute any other spiritual practice you're more comfortable with.

Despite what I've said about the shameful lack of orgies in Voodoo, it is still a sweaty, sexy, primal tradition that engages all the senses. At any Voodoo ceremony in Haiti, drums throb in the humid night air as people dance themselves into trances beneath millions of crystal-clear stars. Without street lights or city glare to distract from this night vision, it is as if you are dancing among the stars. The perfumed aroma of Florida water, dark rum, and *kleren* (raw sugar cane rum), sprayed amongst the crowd by the priest as a healing and cooling balm, mingles with the rich, spicy tang of plantain, curried goat, and yams that you can buy for the equivalent of just a few cents from the traders who line the ceremonial space. Your *moushwa*—the colorful satin headwear worn at a Voodoo dance—will be cool against your skin, and the drums will blend with the songs, laughter, and screams of joy from the crowd.

It's no wonder that in this sensory overload, the spirits of the *lwa*—the angels of Voodoo—want to join in the fun and enter the ritual to offer blessings and perform their magic for the people present.

Like all spirits, the *lwa* are longtime dead, and when they return briefly to life in this way, it's not surprising that healing is not the only thing on their minds. Partying is too! One of these spirits, Baron, the guardian of the cemetery and all its wisdom, is well known as a sexy ghost who wants rum, a fine cigar, and a woman as soon as he shows up in ceremony!

This seems a far cry from the ethereal floatiness we associate with angels (which is what the *lwa* actually are), but if you think about it, there is a spiritual message in their behavior as they get down and dirty: that life is to be lived—fully—and sex is part of that experience. If we deny ourselves these things, well, we may as well be dead, because life becomes a drag.

The *lwa* are our teachers: advisors from the otherworld who pass on their wisdom to a select few. Their teachings might concern healing, foretelling the future, solving disagreements and bringing peace, or ways and techniques for attracting and keeping a lover; there are various specialist and secret societies in Haiti that have received particular teachings from the *lwa* and exist to preserve this wisdom. You will rarely hear about these societies or read about them in books because their knowledge is usually only taught to carefully selected initiates who are invited to join their secret gatherings. One of these societies is the Sisterhood of the Miracles of Night.

The Sisterhood of the Miracles of Night is a woman-only society who are the guardians of sex magic and preserve a goddess-honoring culture that is ancient and pre-Christian in its origins, and which understands the importance of sexual energy for the creation and maintenance of life on earth. The society is led by a "godmother," an older woman whose identity is always kept secret and who is known as *Manman Jenèz* (literally, the Genesis Mother).

As I said earlier, Voodoo is a mix of traditions. At its foundation is African shamanism, but to this, across the years, have been added spiritual practices from many other cultures, including European and Celtic paganism, Jewish Kabbalism, freemasonry, and, of course, Roman Catholicism, so it is not surprising that elements of the Horae traditions of Greece should have become a part of Voodoo as well.

As well as sexual priestesses, the Horae were the "dark goddesses" of time and the seasons, and presided over the revolutions of the heavens and the constellations by which time is measured and the Fates spin their web. Through sex, that is, the whole natural order and the wisdom of the universe can be known. Without it, chaos reigns and life becomes nasty, brutish, and short.

A psychologist friend of mine did some research on this once that showed a correlation between lack of sex; mental, emotional, and physical illness; violence; and warfare. Basically, he said that lack of sexual closeness leads to depression and aggression. To put it in even simpler terms: when we don't get our rocks off, we start throwing rocks at each other, or, at a global level, when we're not "invading each other's countries" in a good way, we invade them in a not-so-good way. When I heard that, I found it difficult to look at George Bush in quite the same way.

So the teachings of the sisterhood are really about making love, not war: world peace through getting a piece. Sex can do this because it's about the freedom to enjoy ourselves, our bodies, and each other without inhibitions or hang-ups, frustrations or judgments, so we get more out of life and are happy and well and sane.

To help you do just that, in this book I'll be introducing you to some of the Voodoo gods of All Things Sexy and showing you a few of the secret techniques of the sisterhood so you can stiffen your sinews and summon up the blood (to paraphrase Shakespeare) even if you've never been that turned on by sex in the past.

I'll also be offering some psychological tips for better flirting, foreplay, and fornication, based on my counseling training and practices, as well as some good old-fashioned sexual common sense.

But if you ask me what this book is *really* about, it's about power—getting your power *back*, that is, from repressive morals that have kept us all suppressed, sexually joyless, and less than juicy for centuries, so you can reconnect with your more healthy, primal, and positively natural self, and experience the art of love as a spiritual practice *and* the most fun you can have with your clothes *off*!

The Goddess Ritual

But first things first. Voodoo ceremonies, rituals, and magic of any kind always begin with an initiation. The word *initiate* means "to start something new," but with spiritual initiation there is also a sense of the sacred. What we are beginning is a new life or a new way of seeing the world, making a commitment to leave the past behind. In our case, we are committing to a new sense of freedom: to be more fully ourselves in our daily lives as well as sexually and spiritually.

Whether initiation involves a long and complex ceremony or a simple prayer to the spirits, it's a formal process that anthropologists say has three stages to it:

1. Putting the everyday world—the world of our habits, conditioning, and hang-ups—behind us

2. Journeying to a new and unfamiliar place

3. Returning to where we began, but in a better way as a result of our journey

T. S. Eliot said it best in his poem "Little Gidding":

We shall not cease from exploration
And the end of all our exploring
Will be to arrive where we started
And know the place for the first time

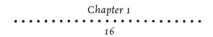
Our journey could mean literally traveling into new and uncharted territory, as the Native Americans do with their vision quests, but always—and more likely—it means a different internal territory: a new frame of mind, so that the concerns of the day and our familiar ways of thinking are left behind and we can enter a deeper state of consciousness. This is what we will do now, because the first step is to become initiates of goddess energy: people who know that there is more to life than we have been told.

This initiation has three elements to it:

1. Relaxing the mind and cleansing the spirit

2. Meeting the Sisters of the Miracles of Night

3. Letting your juices flow

1: Relaxing the Mind and Cleansing the Spirit

If you've read my previous book, you'll know that bathing rituals using special herbs and essences feature heavily in Voodoo. All herbs contain a spirit that is healing, relaxing, or energizing, depending on the nature of the plant and the intention we take to it. Jasmine, for example, is ethereal, relaxing, and brings gifts of insight and prophecy, whereas cayenne is fiery, energetic, and stokes the flames of passion.

In Voodoo, these herbs are also "food" for particular *lwa*, which means that they call specific spirits to us who can help us achieve what we will. Whenever we take one of these baths, there is a three-way magical meeting between the spirits of the plants that we choose, the spirits of the *lwa* that we call, and our own spirit, which is activated through our intention. In this part of the initiation, our intention is simply to relax and cleanse ourselves, so we use herbs that produce this effect and invoke the spirits who can help.

This is the process:

· Run yourself a bath (do not add any soap, bubble bath, or other bathing products).

· To this, add one drop of vanilla extract, a handful of fresh coriander leaves, and three drops of lemon balm (*Melissa officinalis*) aromatherapy oil. (Vanilla is a plant that is often used in spells for love, healing, luck, and for enhanced psychic powers; coriander offers protection and is also used in love spells such as recipes to find an ideal lover; lemon balm is compassionate and gentle.)

· At each corner of the bath, place a white pillar or tealight candle.

· Turn off the lights, light the candles, and then stand naked before the bath, holding in your outstretched hands a handful of red rose petals. Say the following:

> *Erzulie, I call you to bless and protect me,*
> *To energize, relax, and refresh me,*
> *And to hold me in your love and wisdom*
> *So I am safe on the journeys I take*

In Voodoo, Erzulie is the spirit of love, luxury, and abundance, and a protector of children—which, of course, includes you. She is the Voodoo equivalent of Aphrodite, and the sisters, whom we will meet shortly, are her Haitian Horae.

• Sprinkle the rose petals on your bath waters, at the same time saying:

> *These are my gifts to you*
> *In return for your gifts to me*

• Climb into the bath and simply relax. Rub yourself with the petals and coriander leaves, always rubbing downwards to remove negative energies, and pay particular attention to the back of the neck, stomach, elbows, genitals, backs of the knees, and the soles of the feet, where these energies tend to accumulate.

• After fifteen minutes, step out of the bath and pull the plug. Visualize the energies you have removed draining away with the water, then blow out the candles and turn on the lights. (The petals and leaves should be disposed of later by burying them, if possible, at the base of a tree.)

• Dress in red or pink pajamas if you can (if not, clean white pajamas are fine).

- Ideally, there should be no other contact on this day between you and any other living soul. (If you live with three surly cats, however, I'm sure the *lwa* will forgive you.)

2: Meeting the Sisters of the Miracles of Night

The *houngan* (priest) and *mambo* (priestess) of Voodoo are shamans, and, whatever else shamans may be specialists in (plant medicine, for example, or healing rituals), their key approach is the shamanic journey, a special state of consciousness that enables them to commune with the energy (or spirit) of the universe. It is a method for making contact with our guides, recovering energy we have lost, and finding out more about ourselves and our life purpose.

Because we cannot travel to Haiti and meet the sisters in person, we will take a journey like this now in order to meet the sisterhood and pump up our sexual energies. Your visit to the sisters should be taken on the same day as your cleansing bath, so you can greet each other in a spiritually pure state.

To take any shamanic journey, you need to find a time and a place where you can be alone and undisturbed for twenty minutes or so, then dim the lights or cover your eyes, lie down, and make yourself comfortable.

Most shamanic journeys are taken to the sound of a drum. This encourages specific brain-wave patterns to emerge, taking us into a deeper experience of the world in all its fullness. You can drum for yourself or use a drumming tape or CD to guide your journey (see www.thefourgates.com if you need to buy one); both are equally effective.

Expressing your intention—the purpose for your journey—and keeping this in focus is important, because intention is the energy that guides us. So the next thing is to express your intention by putting whatever question or purpose you have into a positive statement of intent. For example, the question "How will I find the sisterhood?" could be expressed positively and definitely as: "My intention on this journey is to meet with the Sisterhood of the Miracles of Night." This statement alerts the spirits to your purpose so they can do the work and answer your question with you.

As soon as the drumming begins, imagine yourself entering a place which takes you down into the earth, such as a well or a cave, and continue through it until you reach your destination: the spirit world where your guides are waiting to help you. Then let your journey unfold as it will.

Haiti is a land of fields, forests, and open spaces, and the sisters always work in natural surroundings. Their magical meetings take place at night, in secret, in the countryside, with trees and plants all around. At their meetings, they stand in a circle with a fire at the center, representing the flames of passion and the energies of sexual union, fifteen women in total.[1] In your mind's eye, see such a scene in front of you, and, closest to the fire, the *Manman Jenèz* (Genesis Mother).

---

1 In Greek tradition, from which this Haitian ritual derives, there were three Horae, the daughters of Zeus (king of the gods) and Themis (the embodiment of divine order), and twelve Hours, the goddesses of the hours of the day. This makes up the fifteen. In Voodoo, the equivalent gods and goddesses are known by different names among the *lwa*. Zeus becomes Loko, for example, and Themis becomes Ayizan. We will meet these spirits later in this book.

Approach the *Manman* and let her welcome you to the circle. As you stand facing the flames, the drums will begin, growing wilder and more frenzied as your body begins to sway and you start to dance to their rhythm. You will be asked to leap the flames of the fire three times: once to release old energies and inhibitions that have been holding you back, once to absorb the heat and passion of the flames into your genitals and lower belly, and once again to seal in your energies of new liberation.

On the third leap, you will stand before the *Manman* again and she will trace four spirals on your skin: at your heart, stomach, genitals, and finally your third eye. This is your initiation into passion, power, creativity, and vision.

You will also be given a nectar to drink—a rich, sugary liquid produced by the flowers to attract honey bees, butterflies, and other life-giving insects to ensure their pollination. This nectar, then, is a potion of sexual power.

As you drink, the drums become quiet and the women start to breathe deeply, at first a rhythmic panting, then building to a chant of "*Pasyon! Pisans! Vizyon! Kouraj!*"—"Passion! Power! Vision! Courage!" The circle becomes quiet again as you finish the drink, and the ritual is complete.

As part of this circle, you may now ask the *Manman*—your godmother—any questions you wish about your sexuality, where you need to let go or embrace new passions, and what your role and purpose may be as a creative and sexual being.

Drumming tapes have a special call-back signal at the end to bring you back to ordinary reality. When you hear this, or when your questions have been answered and you are ready to leave, thank the sisters for accepting you and the *Manman* for her blessings, then turn around and retrace your steps exactly, back to normal awareness.

Be aware of your body and how it feels as you return to ordinary reality. Are you warm from your dance among the flames? What do you feel in your heart, stomach, eyes, and genitals, where new energy was given you? What effects do you sense from the nectar you drank? Move your fingers and toes, feel the floor beneath you, and gently open your eyes.

Make a note, before you forget, of all the things you have seen and experienced, as well as your thoughts and feelings and the answers to your questions, so you have a record you can refer back to. Then sprinkle a little cold water on your face and take a drink. This will help to ground you and bring you back to everyday consciousness.

Watch your dreams and the other messages from your soul for the next few weeks, as the information you have received may still be bubbling away in your unconscious and other revelations may surface.

Watch your feelings and emotions too. A meeting with the sisters is said to stir the passions and, like a kundalini rising, to open you up to "serpent flight": a new awareness of your sexuality.

In short, you may be more turned on than you have been for a while!

3: Letting Your Juices Flow

And now—after all that steamy dancing and drinking the goddess nectar—comes a disappointing part: no sex!

Don't worry, it's not forever! When I became an initiate, I was told that I mustn't have sex after my ceremonies "from full moon to full moon": in other words, no sex for a month.

It could be longer than a month, though, depending on when you took your journey to the sisters. For example, if you had carried out the ritual above on January 3, 2007 (the night of the full moon), you would have to remain celibate until February 2 (the next full moon). If you'd performed the same ritual on January 25, however (the night of the half moon), you would have to wait until March 3 and two full moons had passed in order for you to meet the "full moon to full moon" requirement.

Perhaps I should have told you this before you took your journey so you could get your timing right? Oops. Sorry. (Looks guilty and shuffles feet.)

Still, every cloud has a silver lining … the longer you abstain, the more potent your sexual energy will be, so it's not all bad.

The moon, of course, is the symbol of the feminine and of the goddess to whom you are now connected, so to refrain from sex is to deepen the bond you have formed. This time of abstention also allows your new energies to be integrated and settle, and for the serpent to unfurl so that your kundalini energy can begin its ascent and your body become a fully charged sexual channel.

From full moon to full moon, it is also important to refrain from drinking alcohol and to avoid certain foods. Mainly we follow a vegetarian diet. The reasons for this are that sexual energy is to be used with full consciousness and control, not carelessly wasted because we have drunk too much and fallen into bed with someone—anyone—just for a brief fling, and because sexuality is about life and creativity, not death and destruction, which is why we avoid animal products and meat.

Another aspect of this diet is to take a drink each evening (at nighttime, under the light of the moon) of a special mixture called a dreaming brew. Essentially this is what we in the West would call an aphrodisiac; it's a potion (very tasty, actually) to help us further let go of inhibitions so that sexual energy can flow through us.

The formula for the brew is as follows (the ingredients will be different in Haiti, but these are the equivalents you'll more easily get in the West):

DREAMING BREW

"Nectar": honey, pollen, and royal jelly, blended to a paste (1 tablespoon each). You will find all of these ingredients easily in most health stores.

Plain organic yogurt (6 tablespoons)

Passion fruit (1, peeled and chopped)

Kiwi fruit (1, peeled and sliced)

Fresh lime juice (1 teaspoon)

Ginseng powder (½ teaspoon)

Damiana leaf, powdered (½ teaspoon)

A half-pint of milk, and

A quarter-pint of coconut milk

If this sexual smoothie is too thick for your liking, you can also add mineral water to the consistency you prefer.

Put all the ingredients in a blender and mix until smooth, then drink it immediately while it's good and fresh and yummy! This recipe should give you enough for about two days and will store in the fridge.

As I said before, plants have a particular spirit or vibe to them, and they change the flow of our energies in different ways. The lime in this brew has "drawing in" and attracting qualities and is good for helping to pull sexual energy around the whole body so our nerves are tingling and even our toes are

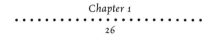
turned on! Ginseng is known for its ability to aid sexual potency, beauty, and healing, and it is used in countless love spells. Damiana is taken to increase magical and sexual energy and is good as a general tonic and as an aphrodisiac. Coconut, meanwhile, is used in protection rituals and in chastity spells. Yes, chastity! The idea is to *feel* your sexual energy, not to blow it, remember!

Together, these herbs will keep you connected to your sexual power, open to goddess energy, and bring you erotic and insightful dreams—so take an interest in what you're dreaming, and record your dreams in a journal until the night of the next full moon.

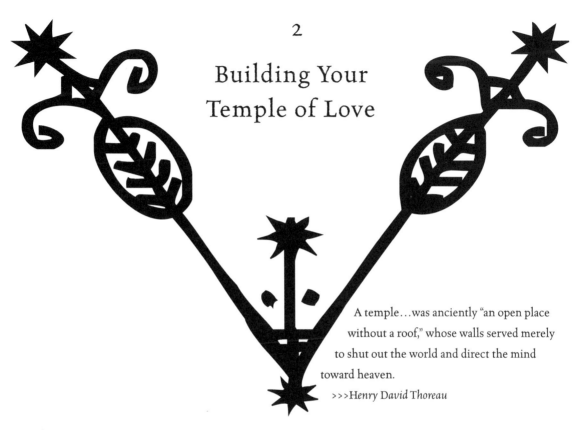

2

Building Your
Temple of Love

A temple…was anciently "an open place without a roof," whose walls served merely to shut out the world and direct the mind toward heaven.

>>>*Henry David Thoreau*

In this chapter, we create our sacred space for love so your sexual explorations channel the right energies to empower and liberate you, and so your intention for love is properly aligned to the goddess.

And then we learn the basics: how to hook a mate to bring back to our temple and play with!

>>>

Every Voodoo ritual takes place in sacred space, whether it's performed in a presidential palace (Voodoo is the official religion of Haiti, and many Haitian presidents have used it to help them win elections), a dingy hut, or a jungle clearing. Ceremonies often take place in the fields, in fact, with no buildings around at all. But it is all still sacred space. Even a shack can be a temple.

When you work with goddess energy, you are working with spirit—the living force of All-That-Is. Creating sacred space is therefore important because it focuses you on the matter at hand and changes the energy of your actions. Sex becomes sacred.

As a relationship counselor, I'm sure that one of the causes of unhappiness in our culture is that we've lost this sacred connection and allowed sex to become something "dirty." Because we think of it as dirty, we act as if it was, and—hey presto!—it becomes dirty, something we do shamefully, a means of "executive stress relief" (which somehow makes it okay) or without thinking too much about it at all. But can a quick fumble in the back row of the cinema really compare with a fully present, fully sexual act where you know that you are a goddess plugged in to the creative powers of the cosmos? I doubt it! Making sex sacred means treating it as sacred.

There's something else about sacred space: no matter where you create it, you take it with you because the sacred itself becomes a part of all you are and all you do. It's your bridge to the spirit world. So even if you do end up in the back of the cinema (and, don't get me wrong, I've nothing against that as a location, per se!), you're still in sacred space and there for the right reasons.

You can create sacred space anywhere (even a cinema) because it's your intention to do so that counts. Given that most of us lead our sex lives in the bedroom, however, I'll show you how to turn that into a temple for love, and you can then adapt the principles for wherever you are at the time.

Turning Your Bedroom into a Temple

There are four steps to creating a sanctuary for love:

1. Prepare the room

2. Prepare the ritual space

3. Call in the gods of All Things Sexy
   through ceremony and intention

4. Then get down to business

1: Preparing the Room

Voodoo is about the magical manipulation of energies, and there are some basics that all practitioners (and, in some cases, modern scientists without a spiritual bone in their bodies) agree you need to take care of before any bedroom becomes a healthy, relaxing, sexually charged space.

For you to feel secure, comfortable, and relaxed so you are in the mood for love, your bedroom should be as far away as possible from the front door of your house. This is a primitive, genetic thing: our prehistoric ancestors never slept near the mouths of their caves because that's exactly where a passing sabertooth would look first in the hope of a snack. Our spirits remember this, but common sense tells us anyway that sex is going to be better when we're not feeling tense and expecting a knock on the door from our neighbor or some other passing predator. So if your bedroom's near the front of the building and you can move it, do it!

If it is and you can't, then make sure there are plenty of lush cushions, drapes, and wall hangings in the room to create a psychological barrier between you and the outside world, and that the room lights are dimmed (like a cave). You'll feel more secure that way, and the bedroom will be cozy and protective. Position your bed as far from the bedroom door as possible, so you can see the door from the bed. This will also give you a sense of added security and allow you to relax.

Where are your windows in relation to your bedroom door? In Voodoo, we know that energy tends to travel in a straight line, so if your door is exactly opposite your window, it will go straight from the door and right out the window (or vice versa) unless you change its flow. Luckily, that's easy enough to prevent, even if you can't change your architecture, by simply ensuring that your windows have adequate drapes so that energy is bounced back into the room, and by making sure that your bed is not between the door and the window so you're not directly in the energy flow. Also make sure that the head of your bed is not too close to the window itself, or your sexual energy will fly out of it too and you'll feel too tired for sex. For the same reason, get a good, strong head-

board so your energies stay in the bed. As an added bonus, it gives you something to hang on to during your mind-blowing orgasms to come.

Beds in general are better made from wood than metal. Wood absorbs energy, giving you a pool of good, loving, sexual energy to lie in, whereas metal acts
like a battery, storing energy and releasing it in unpredictable bursts. I've
known people to get electric shocks from metal-frame beds—which is just
what you don't want when you're whispering sweet nothings!

Beams over the bed can be an energetic headache—literally. They force energy downwards, putting pressure on you and creating a sense of claustropho-
bia or stress. If you've got beams but don't want to totally remodel the house,
paint them so they blend in with the ceiling or drape fabric over them in soothing pastel shades.

Ceiling lamps hanging directly over the bed are a no-no as well. They show
too much and make you feel as if you're auditioning for *X-Factor* instead of cuddling up for sex-factor. Soft, soothing, sensual lighting is much, much better.
Think harem, not scare 'em.

What's under your bed can be as bad as what's above it. A lot of people use
under-the-bed space as a dumping ground for old condom packets; moldy, half-
drunk cups of coffee; squeezed-dry tubes of K-Y Jelly; and acres of other junk
and bad memories.

Get rid of it! Keep the space under the bed clear, and get rid of any clutter
you've thrown there over the years. Imagine yourself meeting your lover-to-be
at a party for the very first time and wearing the stuff you keep under your bed

as your best party outfit, because that's how they'll see you if they look beneath your bed later on. (And don't kid yourself—they *will* look. We all do!)

Your bed space is symbolic of your relationship, your sex life, and your expectations of it. One that's on its last legs, about to collapse, and shored up with a copy of *Sex Tips for Dummies* and a broken vibrator probably says more about you than you want your lover to know!

There's a place and a use for a mirror in every bedroom, but it's not a good idea to have one at the bottom of your bed. Energy is reflected back directly into the bed when you have a mirror facing you, and it'll make you feel tetchy and irritable, so put it in the corner of the room instead, so it helps energy circulate around the room. This will make you both feel more relaxed and as if your performance is not being observed. Only when you know each other a little better is it a good idea to use a mirror as a sex aid.

There is no place at all for a TV in the bedroom! Nothing kills passion as effectively as Jerry Springer or Oprah Winfrey droning on about dysfunctional relationships when you're trying to spread a little love in the world yourself. There's also some scientific research into electrical goods in bedrooms, like radios, TVs, and even clocks, that shows they lead to lethargy, depression, and physical illness. It stands to reason, really, because the more of these you've got around, the bigger the electrical field you're sleeping in. If you wouldn't put your bed under an electrical pylon, don't bring a pylon into your bedroom!

Ladies: beware pinks, frills, "cute" posters of kittens, stuffed toys with "I Wub You" signs hanging from their necks, pictures of ponies, heart-shaped cushions, and other commercial fluff. It'll make you seem clingy, dependent, desperate, and a bit immature given that you're a thirty-year-old cost accountant. Toss them! I don't care to hear about their "sentimental value" or your My Little Pony's "cute ikkle face." If you ever want sex again, get rid of them *now!*

Also beware general dinginess, clothes thrown around the place, half-eaten toast, biscuit crumbs, old socks chucked in a corner, and other detritus. Mess is as bad as fluff. It makes you look like someone who doesn't care—about anything, including sex.

You're a sexual goddess, remember? And you're building a temple here. If you wouldn't expect to find a half-eaten fruit pie and a pair of old panties in a church, you don't want them in your bedroom either.

2: *Preparing the Ritual Space*

But there are some things you *do* want.

In the temples of Aphrodite where the Horae were the priestesses, people who came for healing were met at the gate by fresh young women wearing clean white dresses and flowers in their hair. They were led across spotless floors to cots where clean sheets were placed over them, and they were invited to close their eyes and relax. Flower petals were scattered around them, beautiful perfumes were sprayed in the air, and soothing music was played. By the time it came to sexual healing, those who visited the temple were already feeling better.

In Haiti, the situation's a little different. For a start, it's a third-world country, so there aren't the resources for great, ornate temples. But the principles are the same. Things are kept clean, fresh, and bright. There is a feeling of respect, nurturing, and tenderness toward visitors. Music, perfume, flowers, and other natural things play a part. And all of this is geared toward making guests feel comfortable and invited, and toward clearing a space for energy to move freely so that the sacred is part of all that takes place.

This is the feeling you want to create in your temple too. So, having removed the junk and rearranged your bedroom if you need to, the next thing is to purify the space. You do this in four ways.

1. Firstly, wash the floors (and the walls if you need to) with a mixture of hyacinth, magnolia, and mint in spring water. Hyacinth is the flower of love and protection and also guards against nightmares (and, in this case, nightmare relationships). Magnolia is for fidelity and love. Mint is for affection, and it is loved by all spirits; it is also useful in clearing the mind and increasing your psychic connection during sex.

2. When you've done this, bless the space. Use any words you find appropriate or say out loud this prayer to Erzulie, the Voodoo spirit of love and sexuality:

> *Hold this room in your protection*
> *As a temple for love and true affection;*
> *Give power to the sex that takes place here*
> *And keep the goddess ever near*

3. Now sprinkle a mix of fresh lemon juice and salt across the thresholds of your doors and windows. This seals the room and ensures that unwanted energies can't cross.

4. Finally, use a bell or clap your hands in all corners of the room, from floor to ceiling. Energy gets caught and stagnates in corners, but sound breaks it up and gets it moving again. What you want is a nice circular flow of energy around the room rather than moldy pools that have been hanging around for years, carrying the memories and emotions of all the experiences you've had there—some of which you may not want to remember!

When all that's done, it's time to start rebuilding your temple. Some of the things you might want to include in it are:

Sensual Bedding: Skanky pillows and sheets won't do your sex life any favors. Get yourself new ones in rich, sexy colors and lush fabrics that ooze with lust and positively beg you to stay in bed a little longer.

The Queen of Beds: King-size beds do nothing for intimacy. You can't just turn round, snuggle up, and slip easily into Sunday-morning sex if you have to find your partner first on a mattress the size of a football field. A single bed doesn't cut it either, unless you're both contortionists or sub-size zero and so thin you're practically invisible. Invest in a queen-size bed if you want to get more out of sex.

Do Things in Twos, But Do It Subtly: A single chair, one bedside lamp, bed pillows stacked on one side—all send a message: you're a loner and you're happy that way. If you're serious about sex, invite your lovers in and let them be part of your world: put pillows on both sides of the bed, buy a couple of bedside tables with a lamp on each, get two chairs, a love seat, or a sofa, and angle the chairs toward each other to show that you're ready for love. Do not, however, go crazy here and start buying his and hers pillows, two toothbrushes in pink and blue, or those ghastly "Love Is…" posters that show two gonks (clowns) cuddling up. You've seen Glenn Close in *Fatal Attraction*. Seeing her's enough; there's no need to *become* her. Leave your lover's bunny alone.

Buy Some Appropriate Art: Your bedroom is your temple—your shrine to sex—and the last thing your lover wants to look up and see when he's about to orgasm is a photo of your dear old mom smiling down at him. Looking up in the height of passion and coming face-to-face with a photo of little Dorothy as he's doing her mom can also be a little off-putting. Treat your bedroom as your private retreat, and choose artwork that makes you feel special, sexy, and single—not as if you're having sex in the middle of a family get-together.

Add Some Color: Colors have a big impact on our spirits and, by themselves, can turn us on or off. So, even if you've chosen a color like white as the scheme for your temple, liven it up with splashes of color according to your moods and intentions. Warm shades like reds and golds, and spicy colors like cinnamon, have a sensual feel to them and can juice up your love life considerably. Softer shades like rose and coral create a gentler mood. Bold colors like

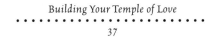
scarlet and burgundy are good for passionate sex and perfect if you're looking for a high-octane fling rather than a serious relationship.

Spread Some Sensual Smells: Investing in an aromatherapy oil burner for the bedroom is a must. Smell is one of our most developed yet subtle senses and is tuned in to the aromas that put us in the mood for love. Once you've got an oil burner, you can experiment with fragrances for passion, oils for unhurried lovemaking, and those which attract lovers and keep them hot to trot! There are a number of these in my book *Va-Va-Voodoo* and a few others here in appendix 2. One you'll definitely want to have around is Temple Oil. This is a blend often used during Voodoo rituals in the West, "temple workings" which contain a sexual element, and magical practices to enhance spiritual and sexual arousal. You can wear this on your skin, apply it to bed sheets, or use it in a burner. This is how you make it:

TEMPLE OIL

Frankincense aromatherapy oil (4 drops)

Rosemary aromatherapy oil (2 drops)

Bay aromatherapy oil (1 drop)

Sandalwood aromatherapy oil (1 drop)

If you're using this in a burner, just add the drops to water. If you want to use it as a massage oil to stimulate the passions and set the mood for sexy encounters, add the ingredients to a cup of almond base oil and mix, then apply to the skin.

3: *Calling in the Gods of All Things Sexy*

Everything we've done so far has been a ritual in itself, which has helped you dress your room and set your intention for sex. Now it's time to empower your space and get it ready for action!

In Voodoo, the way to empower anything is to appeal to the *lwa* for their energy and support. This is done through a ceremony known as *manje-lwa*: feeding the spirits. The one we're about to do is a ceremony for Ogoun and Erzulie.

Erzulie, as you already know, is the Aphrodite-goddess of love, beauty, elegance, poise, grace, luxury, and wealth. She will bring you everything you regard as refined, as well as hot sex, if that's your wish. She is also a very girly spirit and, in return for her help, likes offerings of champagne, chocolates, pastries, roses, makeup, mirrors, and beads.

Ogoun is the warrior-hero of Voodoo, and in his various forms he can appear as a statesman, diplomat, negotiator, teacher, or counselor, as well as a military man. In short, he stands for power, and this is the gift he offers you: sexual power, as well as the power to know yourself, your needs, and to embrace your sexuality fully. Feed him, in return, with rum, cigars, spiced foods, and, if you eat meat, with grilled pork.

Together, Ogoun and Erzulie (who are husband and wife in Voodoo) represent power in love and sex, and power *over* love and sex—which is what you, as a modern goddess, want.

To invoke them, place some of the foods mentioned above on two plates— one for each *lwa*—and put these in the center of your bedroom. In the middle of the plate for Erzulie, light a pink candle (this is her sacred color), and on the plate for Ogoun, light a red candle. Place a photograph of yourself in between the two plates.

Then say these words:

Erzulie, this food is for you
In return for your help and care.
Bring me the perfect lover
To this bed that we will share.
Ogoun, this food is for you
In return for strength and power.
Let goddess energy grow in me
So that my sexual prowess may flower.
Ogoun and Erzulie, this photograph
Is I who make this prayer.
Take the food that is offered
And bring your gifts to me here.

When you have done this, turn around three times in a clockwise direction (the way of increase and attraction), and with the candles burning safely, leave the room.

In Voodoo, it is said that candle flames carry the energy of food to the spirits, and once the candles have fully burned down, your prayers will be heard, the spirits will be fed, and the *lwa* will start working for you.

In the morning, take the candle remains and food and bury them at the base of a tree. Or, if you're an urban Voodoo sex goddess and have no other choice, you can leave them at a crossroads (try to ignore the strange looks you'll get in downtown Manhattan during rush hour).

4: Getting Down to Business

Okay, your work in the bedroom is done and your temple is made, but before you can try it out and test your sexual abilities, you're going to need a sexual partner! Let's go get one—but let's deal with the basics first.

Too often people get excited at the idea of a sexual conquest (or at having sex at all) and don't do their homework first. But if you want the *perfect* lover and the perfect sex, there are some things you need to know—like how to flirt properly.

Perfect sex, despite what Johnny Rotten had to say about it, is not just three minutes of squelching noises and flapping around like landed cod; it's a whole ritual, and 90 percent is mind power, not sexual athletics. The best lovers in the world—and all sexual goddesses—know how to get into their lover's minds before they get into their pants, because even a gesture, a look, or a word can have an explosive sexual impact before any physical contact takes place.

So here's my guide to successful flirting, which you can use, by the way—and which adds a big dollop of spice to any relationship—even if you've been married for thirty years.

How to Flirt like a Goddess

Flirting is a basic human instinct found in all cultures of the world (which is not surprising, really, because without some way of attracting a partner and getting down to sex, the human race wouldn't be here), but in Haiti it is practically an art form, and one of the ways to measure the magical power of a *houngan* or *mambo* is by the number of sexual partners and devoted followers they have. In Haiti it is not considered a crime to use the sexual powers that God has given us in this way; to not do so, in fact, would be the crime, as well as be wholly unnatural.

Even though flirting is universal, instinctive, and natural, goddesses aren't helped by the fact that a lot of men are stupid. Research shows, for example, that men find it quite hard to gauge a woman's body language, which flirting relies upon, and can even mistake a come-on for a brush-off. Once again, it's down to women to save the species by perfecting the art of flirting so even men can see it for what it is!

To give you an edge in this, before you even leave the house, I want to offer you a secret weapon: the recipe for a magical Voodoo perfume called a *sant*. This word simply translates as "scent" so it hides the power of this potion, which is to change your energy so you become incredibly attractive to the opposite sex (or to your own, if that is your preference).

In Haiti, it is said that these perfumes can make anyone fall hopelessly in love with you by making your spirit radiant and your sexual energies intense. And all you need do is wear them as you would any perfume.

Sants are combinations of magical herbs, and there are many different for-mulae, each of which is a guarded secret of a particular *houngan* or *mambo*, and they are all said to be equally effective. Rather than give you one recipe, there-fore, in the chart opposite I've listed the herb that is used in Haiti, its English or American equivalent, and others that could be used instead or as well, based on European Voodoo practices. From this, you can make up your own perfumes and see which you prefer and which works best for you.

You can use fresh herbs or aromatherapy oils to create your recipes. Work around the main ingredient (i.e., those in the second column) so this becomes your base, and add to this a little of the others that interest you, so that the ratio of the main ingredient to the others is about 3:1. If you use fresh herbs, take a little of each and add them to alcohol (vodka is good for this, as it is colorless and odorless). If you use aromatherapy oils, you can simply drop them into a bottle containing a base oil of sunflower.

Either way, once the blend is made, take it to your temple and offer it to the four directions, asking the spirits of love and power, Erzulie and Ogoun, to bless it and make it potent. Feed the spirits in return and leave the bottle in their care for nine days.

Haitian Name	English Name	European Voodoo Alternatives	What it Does
Amwaz	Motherwort	Carnation, Ginger, Rowan	Increases spiritual power and sexual allure
Bonbonyen	Lemon Verbena	Allspice, Daffodil, Fern, Rose, Violet	Brings luck in love
Lalwa	Aloe Vera	Almond, Basil, Bergamot, Jasmine	Bathes you in love and protection
Melon dlo	Watermelon	Honeysuckle, Peppermint, Thyme, Lavender, Passionflower	Improves powers of empathy and intuition, and balances the emotions
Shoublak	Hibiscus	Pansy, Rose, Willow	Draws love
Sitwonnel	Lemongrass	Licorice, Patchouli	Increases lust and makes others lust after you
Vanille	Vanilla	Cardamom, Coriander, Hyacinth	Makes you irresistible to others
Zoran'y	Sweet Orange	Flax, Ginseng	Increases beauty

After this, you can use the oil directly by applying it to your skin, or, if you are using fresh herbs in vodka, strain the mixture and add a little water to dilute it, then decant it into an atomizer so you can use it as a spray.

Recipes I have enjoyed using (with some success) include lemon verbena with bergamot and jasmine to develop a loving connection to others. This also gives me protection so my outrageous flirting does not get me into trouble. I also like vanilla, coriander, and ginseng, which makes me feel beautiful, fresh, and irresistible.

One tip I can offer, though, as you make up your blends, is that some research done in the UK into the attractive power of fragrances found that the number one aroma men go for is … wait for it … licorice. It probably reminds them of childhood and makes them feel safe, even if they are in the presence of a vamp! So you may want to add a hint of licorice to your blends.

Now that you have your secret fragrant flirting weapon, here are a few facts about the art of the flirt to give you an idea of how to proceed.

FIRST IMPRESSIONS DO MATTER

- We form opinions of each other within 90 seconds of meeting
- 55 percent of first impressions come from body language
- 38 percent are from tone of voice
- Only 7 percent of your impact comes from what you say

quickie
SEX
Facts!

As with all magic, the first thing in flirting is to get your intention right. A good flirt isn't there to play games or show off, but to give someone a signal. So the idea is to show an interest in them, not to prove to yourself that you know a bunch of bed-hopping tricks (even if that is what I'm about to teach you)!

Flirting is mostly about what you do, not what you say. In fact, words have little to do with it, because first impressions are based on body language, then tone of voice, and only then what we say. Words themselves are ambiguous. Your "Hi, how are you doing?" could mean anything from "Oh God, it's that nerd from the office" to "Wow! You're a sex god and I want you now!" It's how you say it that counts. So because it's all in the body, here's what to do:

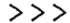

KNOW WHO TO FLIRT WITH

- **People between 35–44 are the world's biggest flirts**
- **50 percent in this age range say it's their "favorite hobby"!**
- **70 percent of people in long-term relationships still flirt with strangers; they say it gives them the hots for their regular partner (a likely story?)**

Chapter 2

Make Eye Contact

In most flirt manuals, eye contact is about showing him you're interested, and you can signal this even across a crowded bar by holding his gaze for just over a second (but no longer). People tend to look away in less than a second when we meet their eyes, so if we hold their gaze for longer it signals a definite interest.

In Voodoo, we don't just flutter our eyes, though; we use them as a channel for sexual energy. It's well known in Voodoo that the sex organs have their own *djab*, or spirit, and that the eyes allow this spirit to take flight from the body and enter the body of another. So when you see someone you like the look of, hold their gaze—and during that intimate little-over-a-second, take your inner attention to your genitals and scoop up some of the energy you find there, then flick it out through your eyes and in through theirs. This subtle gesture is known as an *expedition*— the sending of a spirit or intention—and it should produce a definite effect!

Once you've hooked through looks and got into a conversation, you can repeat this gesture so your *djab* goes to work on his energies. Hold his attention by looking at him as he talks, in glances of between one and seven seconds (again, no more). Five to seven seconds is the optimum glance time for developing intimacy, but don't overdo it: the most common mistake in flirting is too much eye contact, which makes the other person nervous. When you look him directly in the eyes, his body produces chemicals like those released when he's in love. It's automatic. He just can't stop himself.

Your main Voodoo trick, however, is your *sant*. This magical perfume also has its own spirit, which has been charged and fed to draw lovers toward you, and the longer you can keep him in your presence, the greater the effect it will have. The flirting techniques that follow, therefore, have one aim in common: to hold on to him while your Voodoo does its work!

Move a Little Closer (But Not Too Close)

We carry our comfort zones with us. Our "social zone" (minimum safe distance from somebody else) is about four feet around us; our "personal zone" (the bit we like to keep to ourselves) is about four feet to eighteen inches from the body. After that, you're into the "intimate zone" (only for lovers and close friends and family). Here's how you use this information …

Having made eye contact and started the chat-up process, begin to move a little closer, going through the four-foot barrier if you sense it's okay. If it's not, you'll be met with a few barrier signals, like crossed legs, folded arms, and a body angled away from you. If you see any of these, back off quickly but subtly, and try again a little later. If you get an okay, however, keep moving in, slowly but surely, until you're in his personal zone. If you still get no signals to back off, chances are you could be ending the evening in each other's intimate zones.

Give the Right Signals

Watch his posture for tell-tale signs, and try to send the right ones with your own. Some examples:

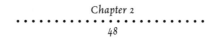
We tilt our heads to one side when we fancy the person we're talking to. If you get the opposite signal, with his head turned toward you and his body angled away, you're going to have to work a lot harder.

Leaning backwards or supporting the head on one hand are signs of boredom. Hair-flipping, head-tossing, and fiddling with the hair, however (especially by women), are positive unconscious gestures that demonstrate sexual interest.

Another good sign is what we psychologists call "postural echo." This is when the person you're talking to unconsciously adopts a posture similar to yours. You can use this deliberately (but subtly) to create a better connection. Sip your drink when he picks up his, or move your hand to the bar when he looks around for the waiter (you get the idea).

Real and False Smiles

If someone smiles at you, it generally means he finds you attractive—but not always. So when is a smile not a smile? There are four ways of telling the difference:

1. Real smiles produce wrinkles around the eyes; false ones don't

2. Real smiles cover the whole face; forced smiles don't

3. Real smiles turn up at appropriate moments in the conversation; false smiles don't look right and appear stiff

4. Real smiles are fleeting and frequent; manufactured ones are held longer

Use Your Voice: What to Say and When

Signs of attraction have more to do with his tone of voice than the words he uses. If your guy gives you a deep, drawn-out "Hello," rising at the end like he's asking you a question, it's a good sign (the question he's really asking, by the way, is "Would you like to sleep with me?"). On the other hand, if you get a short, high-pitched squeak of a "Hello," either you're going to have to work a whole lot harder or you just scared him half to death.

Watch how you speak as well. A dull, monotone delivery with no variation in pitch, pace, or tone will make you seem boring, but go too far the other way (loud, fast, and shrill) and you'll just sound overbearing. Go for the mid-range. Add a bit of moderation, vary your pace, and change your rhythm once in a while.

Forget the legendary "opening line" as well. Overblown chat-up lines and cheese like "Did it hurt when you fell from heaven?" *sound* like obvious come-ons, and using them makes it seem like you lack confidence and self-esteem. The best opener, believe it or not, is simply "Hello."

Keep your conversation open to invite further dialog. There's a difference, for example, between "What do you think of the party?" and "This party really sucks, doesn't it?" The former encourages a response, while the latter will get you (at best) a yes or a no answer (and maybe a slap round the face if you've used it on the host). If you are not sure of the difference between open and closed questions, open-ended chat lines begin with Who, What, When, Where, How, or Why.

What you talk about is also important. Negativity is a big turn-off. Complaints, self-interest, banal comments, and a lack of enthusiasm don't do it for most people. Compliments, on the other hand, work a treat. Research shows that the best compliments use the word "you" in 75 percent of cases and the word "nice" in 25 percent. "That's a really nice color on you" or "Your hair looks nice" is as good as anything, as long as it's said with sincerity.

Use your sense of humor as well. Just about every lonely hearts ad asks for a GSOH (good sense of humor), and studies show that people who genuinely *do* have a GSOH are seen as more likeable and sexy. The best humor in flirting is playful teasing. This allows both of you to increase the "personal" content of your conversation, while keeping the tone nonthreatening. Men really like banter because it's similar to the ribbing they take part in with friends, so it feels safe to them.

And Finally: Say Farewell, Not Goodbye (And Make Sure You Go for the Close)

Your best shots at flirting will usually be quick encounters in public places like bars, where there are other people around—so you're up against a deadline if you're looking to take things further. Your approach to the ending is crucial because it determines what (if anything) happens next.

You want a "closer" that gives you the chance to meet again. Simple, straightforward honesty is usually the best policy, so take your courage in hand and just ask. "Would you like to meet me for lunch next week?" or something like that is fine as long as it's clear and not stumbling or awkward. Remember: you are a goddess and you have nothing to fear!

What to expect next depends on how well you've followed the rules, but some indications are these:

- Men who are looking for a fling are five times more likely to text you straight after you've flirted together

- If they're looking for a more serious relationship, however, they'll leave it a day or two

- 75 percent call within two days of the first date, so if they haven't contacted you at all by the end of the week, just forget it and move on. You're a goddess, after all, and the world is your aphrodisiac oyster!

And, as a goddess, let's not forget why you're flirting in the first place: because sex is your healing method of choice. So now there's something else we must do: ensure that this healing channel is open.

The Marriage of Ogoun and Erzulie

A Voodoo "marriage ceremony" between power and love
to reclaim our bodies as sacred channels

In Voodoo, sex is an expression of power (*ashe*): the creative force for love and healing that permeates the entire universe. The *lwa* who best represent this blending of love and power are the husband-and-wife team of Ogoun and Erzulie.

Our bodies are also sacred channels, the temples for our souls. The vagina represents the gateway, the door to the stars, through which the traveler may pass into realms of the *lwa* and infinite mystery. The penis represents this traveler, the warrior-explorer (Ogoun) who passes through the portal of sexual power (represented by Erzulie) to discover new worlds and return with gifts and blessings. We can see some of this symbolism in *vevers*, the mystical signs used for each of these *lwa*.

The first is for Erzulie, and alongside it is a diagram of the vagina and ovaries. There are obvious similarities, not least in the heartlike shape of each and the M shape at their centers.

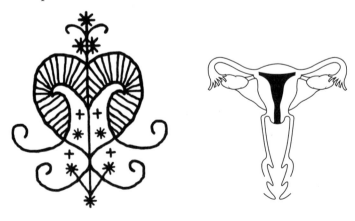

The M in the *vever* stands for *manman* (mother), but also for *maji* (magic) and *mitan* (heart): "the magical heart of the mother." At the center of every Voodoo *peristyle* (church) in Haiti, there is also a central post called the *porteau mitan* (gateway of the heart), down which the spirits descend from Gine (the spirit world) to bring gifts of healing, insight, divination, and messages from the spirit universe—like they were being born anew every time. The vagina, then, is the gateway for love and blessings, and every woman, by simply having one, *is* the gateway between worlds.

The *vever* below is for Ogoun, and alongside it is a diagram of the penis. Again, note the similarities.

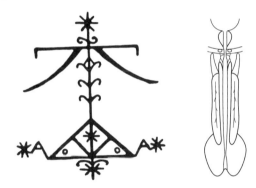

The triangle at the base of the *vever* (corresponding to the testes in the image on the right) is a symbolic cannon, because Ogoun is a man of war. The cannon is a device from which shots are fired. In Haiti, as in most parts of the world, the penis is known colloquially as a "weapon" (*zam*) and to orgasm is to "shoot." Once shot, the cannonball/sperm is sent into space to make its own way.

The penis and the life-giving sperm it contains is the "traveler between worlds." Should it be successful in its journey and reach the egg, the baby that is created is brought into this world from the land of the spirits (*les invisibles*) through the gateway that is the mother.

To bring these two great forces together—male and female, traveler and gateway, penis and vagina, sperm and egg—is to create a new sacred energy. This is done when any baby is made and also occurs naturally in hermaphrodites, who, in Haiti, as in many shamanic cultures, are revered as seers and mystics because they automatically walk in both worlds.

Bringing these forces—Ogoun and Erzulie—together, then, reminds us of our sacred power and sexual duties. The *maryaj-lwa* (marriage to the spirits) is one way of doing so.

In Haiti, *maryaj-lwa* is an actual marriage between a man or woman and the *lwa* he or she has chosen as a partner. The *houngan* will arrange a wedding ceremony, with champagne, cake, and rings to be exchanged, and then call on the spirit to appear through its possession of someone present who acts as a volunteer. The (human) bride and (spirit) groom—or vice versa—make their vows to each other as a union of the worlds. The spirit-husband agrees to protect and take care of his wife and imbue her with his power from that day forth, while she provides the gateway through which he may enter the physical world.

You can do something like that now too by opening yourself to new power through a symbolic gesture in the form of a journey like the one we took in the last chapter.

Go to your temple, lie on your bed, and close your eyes. Now allow your mind to drift and an image to form of a beautiful woman (Erzulie) who embodies all there is to know about love, and a handsome, strong, and distinguished man (Ogoun) who represents all there is to know about power, charisma, and ultimate cool. See them both standing there, as husband and wife, symbolizing love and power in its fullness. Watch as they make love, delighting in each other's bodies; watch as Erzulie's belly begins to swell and her man watches over her as their baby starts to grow; watch as the union of love and power, the holy child, is born.

At this moment, step forward and ask the mother and father of the sacred if you may hold this child. As you do so, allow the baby to bless you through its breath, passing on some of its essence and energy to you so you, too, become love and power, a sacred channel for the divine.

You may feel it in your body or your soul as this transference of power takes place. You may also catch flashes of a symbol of some kind, a *vever* just for you, which symbolizes your connection to All-That-Is, the kind and infinite force that is the goddess energy of the universe, known in Voodoo as *Bondye* (good god).

Open your eyes when you're ready, and write down the details of your journey, then draw your *vever* of love and power. Sleep with it next to you. It's something to keep in your temple.

3

How to Kiss like a Pro (And Other Things Your Body Can Do)

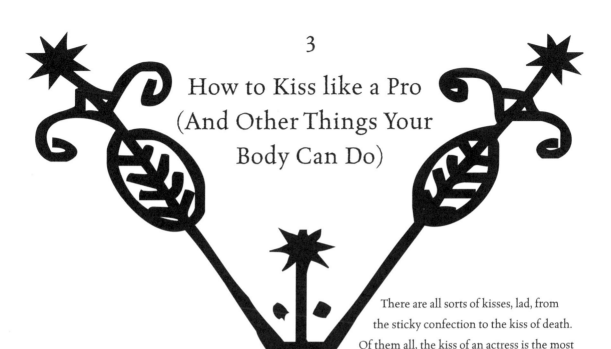

There are all sorts of kisses, lad, from the sticky confection to the kiss of death. Of them all, the kiss of an actress is the most unnerving. How can we tell if she means it or if she's just practicing?

>>>*Ruth Gordon*

In this chapter we come to grips with the arts of love—how to kiss, how to explore each other's bodies—and we learn some of the Tantric secrets of Voodoo: using the body's "nectars" in love spells for magical success, and how to make sex go on forever ("to infinity and beyond!").

Okay, everyone knows how to kiss. You put your lips together and make like you're chewing a sweet, right?

Not exactly. There are hundreds of ways to kiss (the *Kama Sutra* lists over 250) and different effects any kiss can create. We haven't got space for all 250 here (and you'd never remember them anyway), but I'll give you a few ideas you can try in just one minute. First, though, what's kissing all about?

Kissing is an act of trust, nurturing, and love. In some tribal traditions from which Voodoo stems, it's still quite common for mothers to wean their children from the breast and onto solid foods by chewing the food first and then passing it to the child mouth-to-mouth. This is the most natural thing in the world and we also see it in the animal kingdom, like when birds feed their young. According to anthropologists, this is probably the origin of kissing.

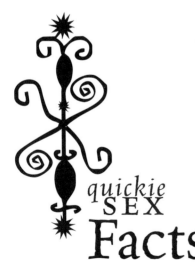

ADDICTED TO LOVE?

- During a passionate smacker, the body produces oxytocin, a chemical associated with happiness, faithfulness—and addiction. That's how you keep him faithful!

- Every kiss burns 26 calories a minute—as good as an aerobic workout!

- 60 percent of women say that kissing is more fun than sex—so it pays to perfect the art!

But it's also true that kissing is about simple pleasure. There are more than 100,000 nerve endings in your lips (by contrast, the clitoris has 8,000—and you know how good that feels), each one capable of giving you a pleasurable little shock like a tiny orgasm when a tongue is run sensuously over it.

In some of the sisterhood's secret teachings, it is known that the nerves of the lips run directly to the nipples—a major erogenous zone for men and women. Furthermore, the nerves in a woman's upper lip link via a hidden pathway to her clitoris, while the nerves on a man's lower lip go to his penis. The same knowledge turns up in little-seen ancient Tantric texts, by the way, so perhaps this is universal but hidden sexual and spiritual information. Either way, it may account for the fact, discovered by sex researchers, that some people (mainly women) can orgasm from kissing alone. A very underrated sexual skill, the kiss.

And it is actually one of the simplest to learn. If you want to be an excellent kisser and go for the orgasm-by-kiss-alone, just study your partner!

Relax your mouth and don't do anything. Then ask *him* to demonstrate his perfect kiss on you. Lie back and enjoy it and, as you do, make a mental note of the details: how long the kiss lasts, how he holds you at the time (there's more than just lip action in kissing), if—and how deeply—he thrusts his tongue into your mouth, how juicy he likes his kisses, and so on. Then go away and practice in private, using those finest of teenage sex aids, the back of your hand or your pillow!

In no time at all, you'll be his favorite kisser—and all you're actually doing is letting him kiss himself.

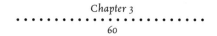
To kick-start (or should that be kiss-start?) your research process, here are a few techniques to try:

The Lick, Suck, and Nibble

Before your lips touch your partner's lips, run the tip of your tongue around your partner's lips, starting at the top left if you're kissing a guy and completing a circle counter-clockwise (or from bottom right if you're kissing a girl, completing the circle in a clockwise direction). This activates the nerves that lead directly to the genitals.

Try varying the amount of tongue as well, so you make your kisses wetter and more earthy, or use the tip to gently flick his lips with a butterfly movement. If you're groin-to-groin as you kiss, you should notice an effect from your man within seconds!

The Guppy

Vary the rhythm and depth of your kiss by sucking gently on his lower lip (or her upper lip) like a guppy sucking on the wall of a fish tank, or by *very gently* pulling on your partner's lip with your teeth, for a truly primal kiss.

The Frenchie

This is a whole-body kiss, so press yourself against your partner as your lips meet, pushing your groin ever-so-slightly into his. Run your fingers through his hair, paying particular attention to the hairline at the base of his neck (this is one of the body's most erotic erogenous zones), where you can also stroke and tickle gently. As the kiss hots up, let your hands slide seductively down his back to grip his bottom, pulling his groin into yours.

Use your tongue to explore the inside of his mouth as well, circling his tongue with yours and giving little flicks to the inside of his upper lip to encourage him to use his tongue in your mouth. Pull away from each other's lips—but not too far!—from time to time so that only your tongues meet and circle each other, then come back together by sucking his tongue into your mouth.

So it doesn't get too hot, sloppy, and steamy, control the pace with little closed-mouthed kisses from time to time, which hardly touch the lips at all. Then build up again to more frenetic kissing and slow down once more, so you never quite reach a climax and keep your lover right on the edge.

Elemental Kissing

Here are a couple of techniques you can try when you're past the first date and things are getting a bit more experimental.

Air kissing is a technique taught by the sisterhood that is about using the breath to stimulate your partner. Begin by blowing a soft current of air over and across his lips, as if you were licking them with your tongue. To him it feels like warm chiffon being run gently over all those sensitive nerve endings in his lips. Vary your action by introducing little pecks and tongue flicks before your lips finally meet.

Water kissing is definitely not one for the first date—or the cocktail lounge, for that matter! With this kiss, you pass an ice cube back and forth between your mouths, using your tongues to make the exchange. This creates a delicious combination of heat and cold and will also make your tongues more sensitive. As the ice cube melts, so do you!

To state the obvious: it's not always a good idea to go through all of these techniques at once, or you'll seem like a confused lip gymnast! Find your own rhythm, pace, likes and dislikes, then practice—and play!

If the time and the space are right, all of this lip action can really only go one way: into the bedroom. And there are some things you should know when you get there.

In the Zone

Erogenous zones are areas of the body that, like the lips, offer us a luscious number of nerve endings to play with, all of which, in one way or another, end up at the genitals. Knowing your way around them gives you a map of your lover's body and will earn you a reputation as a sexual goddess, as well as his undying love and appreciation!

Knowing the body—yours as well as his (and literally from top to bottom)—is an essential part of sex and a developed skill in Haiti, where massage and attention to the body's trigger points are often an important part of Voodoo healing. Knowing the body also means you know what *you* like and can ask for it (which helps your lover to relax by turning sex into less of a guessing game) and also that you have a good idea of what will do it for him as well. So, as we go through the erogenous zones below, explore them for yourself by touching your body there and seeing how they feel to you.

The Head

As you're a woman, you probably fiddle with your hair a lot. Ever wondered why? Because it feels good! Having your hair brushed, fussed with, and tended to can be a very sensual experience. Why do you think women spend so much time and money at the hairdressers every week?

It's exactly the same for men, but as men aren't into personal grooming as much as the opposite sex, they probably haven't discovered the exquisite pleasure they can get from it. But run your fingers through his hair or brush your fingers over it as you kiss him, and he'll soon be putty in your hands—and then he'll know why you spend Saturday afternoons with the stylist while he's watching football!

The Neck

The neck in general is one of our sexual hotspots, and the back of the neck, where the hairline ends, is even hotter. Stroking, tickling, and brushing your fingertips over it can have a grown man (or woman) panting and whimpering in your arms if you do it right.

But don't forget the rest of the neck. Working your way around it, planting little kisses, licks, and hot breath on the skin, works wonders. Just don't overdo the hickies (if you need to do them at all). Some people enjoy them at the time,

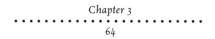
but won't thank you for them later because of the way they look, the impression they give to others ("You don't get those standing up!" as we used to say in the school yard), and because they'll have to wear high collars and turtlenecks for a week (which is not a great look for the beach).

The Ears

There are sensitive nerve endings in and around the ears, and kissing, stroking, blowing, and nibbling there is a turn-on for most people. Make a little noise while you're at it as well. Little moans and whimpers are half the fun of ear play.

The Lips

I've already talked about these and the thousands of nerve endings there that connect directly to your genitals, so let me just add this: in surveys, the biggest desire of people in long-term relationships is more kissing. It's the first sexual thing we do with each other and the first thing to go when we've been seeing each other awhile—and that's a big mistake!

The Small of the Back

The back is not only full of juicy nerve endings, it's a part of the body where stresses tend to accumulate. Surprising your lover with a massage using the palm of your hand or stroking it with your fingertips (or better still, your tongue) is a guaranteed crowd-pleaser during unhurried sex, and the less stress he feels, the better he'll appreciate the main event.

The Buttocks and Anus

There's no getting away from it: men and women both like attention to their buttocks. A light touch there can send shivers up the spine, and, because they're big muscles, the buttocks can take a lot of kneading and squeezing too, and licking around and between them can be incredibly arousing. They're also a good stopping-off point if you're working your way down to your final destination.

The anus has a lot of nerve endings and is very sensitive. Some people are squeamish about what they see as "ass play," but stimulating this area with fingers or tongue ("rimming"), or inserting a finger into a willing partner, can bring pleasure to you both. Give it a try and make up your own mind.

The Calves

Try running your fingers lightly down the outside of your calves, from just below the knee to just above the ankle, and you'll experience a delicious sensation partway between tickling and orgasm. Spend some time on this area, exploring the backs of your knees as well, and then imagine the effects you'll have on him!

The Feet and Toes

Licking around—and especially between—the toes will also give him the part-tickle, part-orgasm experience! The toes are more sensitive than the rest of the foot, but don't let them grab all your attention: brushing your hair over the instep and the soul of the foot can produce dramatic and sensual effects. Try "stroking" the whole foot with your hair first, then using the flat of your tongue on the top of them and working your way down to and around the toes. Use a firmer tongue to push between the toes and lick around them—and watch him wriggle in ecstasy!

And now we work our way back up the body, this time from the front:

The Perineum

The perineum is the area between the vagina and anus (or, on a man, between the testicles and anus). It's incredibly soft and sensitive, and made from tissue similar to the vaginal lips, so there are a lot of nerve endings there. Strangely enough, though, it's an area often overlooked during sex play, but put your explorer's cap on and take an adventure—light touches at first, followed by stroking and tickling—and you'll find it's well worth the visit!

The Clitoris

There used to be a time when most women would say they didn't know where their clitoris was (ask your granny)—and most men genuinely didn't (ask your mother). I hope that's changed now, but on the off-chance that anyone is still in the dark about this: the clitoris is the lumpy bit at the top of the vagina, nestled between the labia.

Women differ about the amount of pressure they like on their clitoris during petting, so experiment using different levels of pressure, rhythms, and ways of touching. Wet your finger to simulate the feeling of oral sex and see how you like this "tongue" to move as well.

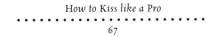
The Breasts and Nipples

Men have breasts and nipples as well as women, and they're a turn-on for both sexes. Indirect stimulation of the nipples, working around them, stroking and kneading the breast, or rubbing and flicking the nipples is generally best until they become hard and aroused. After that a firmer touch is fine, and some women love having their nipples pinched and tweaked or pulled and stretched with a fair bit of vigor.

This is one erogenous zone where women (and men) with smaller breasts have one over on their bigger-busted rivals, because all breasts and nipples have exactly the same number of nerve endings, so a woman with smaller breasts actually gets more thrills per inch.

The Glans (Head of the Penis) and Testicles

The glans is the purple, helmet-shaped knob at the top of the penis. The most sensitive part is the base of the glans and especially its underside, where the head makes an inverted V (for Voodoo) shape. This V is the ending of one of the secret energy pathways that the sisterhood teach is connected to the lips. Gently rubbing (or even better, licking) along the glans, then following the line of the V up to the tip of the penis, will drive any man wild, particularly if you then pop the head in your mouth and suck gently.

The testicles live in the sack of flesh beneath the penis called the scrotum. This is a soft spot and highly sensitive. Treat it gently, stroking and cupping the testicles with your hand, or licking and nibbling along the underside, then taking one or both testicles in your mouth and making a soft "mmm" sound so your lips vibrate as your tongue laps around them. Vary this with attention to the penis itself, and your man will be convinced that you've wafted into his life from paradise (which, of course, as a sexual goddess, you have)!

Of all the erogenous zones, the woman's vagina and clitoris and the man's penis and testicles are the jackpot areas and the places you'll inevitably get to if sex is what you're aiming for, so let's take a good look at these.

Getting to Know You, Part 1: Finding Your Way Around a Penis

The average penis size, no matter what you've heard or the boasts you've had to listen to, is less than six inches in length (about 5–5.9 inches, to be exact) and 4.85 inches in circumference when erect. Flaccid, it's a whole lot smaller.

It's said that there are two types of penises: *showers*, which are relatively big in the flaccid state, and *growers*, which are nothing to write home about until they get erect and may then lead to a raised eyebrow or two. Either way, it doesn't make much difference: there aren't many penises longer than six inches when they're dressed for business and, in any case, it's not what they look like, but what *you*, as a goddess, *can help them to do* that matters. So get yourself a carrot and try the following moves.

There's more than one way to skin a rabbit, as we say in England, and more than one way to handle a penis, but always, always, the first rule is to be *gentle*! You're not holding a hockey stick.

The Grip Stroke

Begin by lightly gripping the penis and sliding your hand up and down from top (just beneath the glans) to bottom. Then gently pull down the foreskin (if he's got one—in Europe he probably will, in America it's less common) and slide your fingers to the base, choosing points along the way and squeezing rhythmically on both sides as you go.

Bell Ringing

Start with one hand lightly grasping the top of the penis and stroke from top to bottom, then release. As you do so, bring your other hand to the top and repeat, so it becomes a two-handed, continual motion.

The Twister

With one of your hands, pull downwards while applying a gentle corkscrewing motion to the top of the penis with the other. This is the one you'll see porn actresses doing in the movies. It looks fancy but doesn't give that much extra pleasure to your man, so it depends on the effect you're after.

Opening the Door

Slowly and gently rotate your hand round the head of his penis like you're turning an oily doorknob. Repeat and reverse direction once in a while. This move is definitely improved by using lubricant.

Doing It His Way

This is the technique that'll make you famous if you do it right. First, ask yourself this question: who is the expert on his penis? He is, of course: he's probably pulling it himself half a dozen times a week, according to the figures on male masturbation, and he may have spent thirty years doing it. So, as near as you can, you want to do what he does to make himself happy.

With most men, that's taking the penis in two hands at the top with the index and middle fingers, applying slightly more pressure at that inverted V of the glans I mentioned earlier. The thumbs line up on the other side of the penis and exert light pressure too, while the other fingers wrap around the shaft to simulate a vagina. Now make small movements, of about an inch or two, down the shaft and up again, at a rhythm of about 200 beats per minute. Vary the pressure slightly as you go, and speed up when his breath gets shallower and he gets a weird look on his face. And that's all there is to it! Trust me: this one's got a 100 percent hit rate!

quickie
SEX
Facts!

LUST SIGNS IN MEN

- **If he's into you, you'll know! Men get erect within 30 seconds of sexual stimulation**
- **60 percent of men's nipples harden when they're turned on**
- **25 percent of men flush when they're excited—the skin reddens on the stomach and spreads to the chest, face, and neck**

Getting to Know You, Part 2:
Finding Your Way Around a Vagina

This is the information your lover needs to know (some women might not know all of this either), so be sure to leave this section lying open "by accident" when he's around—or, better yet, work through it together.

The average vagina is one inch in diameter and four inches deep, the vulva entering the body at a 45-degree angle, with the cervix at the head of this tube. About two inches in, on the top side, is the infamous G-spot, a bundle of nerves that, when stimulated, can lead to the legendary vaginal orgasm.

To find your G-spot, insert your finger approximately three inches into your vagina and hook it backwards. Move it with a small circle at this point and explore a little. It should feel very nice indeed!

The vagina's other hotspot is the clitoris (or clit), which contains around 8,000 nerve endings—the greatest concentration in either the male or female body, and all it's there for is to make you feel good! But there's even better news …

The part of the clitoris you can see is the clitoral hood, but the clitoris is also a two- to four-centimeter path of nerves that extends back toward the anus, making the clitoris nine centimeters long in total and available for pleasure all the way!

Men, here's how you use this information:

Labia Massage

Some men go straight for the clitoris or, worse still, stick a finger or two into the vagina as soon as they have your pants off. But there's a lot more pleasure to be had—and to be got and given—before you get to that point. Begin, instead, with light stroking around her inner thighs, barely touching the skin. Don't go much further until her pelvis begins to arch upwards. At this point she can't help herself; she's inviting you in. Respond by placing your hand over her labia, fingers pointing toward her anus, and gently stroking upwards. Explore the inner and outer lips of her vagina with your fingers, but don't put your fingers inside her yet. Keep her hot!

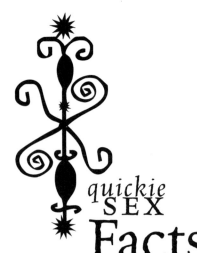

LUST SIGNS IN WOMEN
- Women can take up to 45 minutes to orgasm, so you're going to have to work for it, men!
- The breasts swell by 20 percent and the nipples harden when a woman's turned on
- 75 percent of women flush when they're excited—the skin reddens at the throat, then the abdomen, and spreads to the breasts

In and Out

When she's wet from the attention you've given her, insert one, then two fingers into her vagina (middle finger first), and rest your thumb on her clitoris. Now you can rub your fingers across her G-spot while your thumb massages her clitoris, a combination that will drive her wild.

Cervical Massage

The cervix is in the upper part of the vagina and feels like a little dome of tissue with a small indentation in the middle. Now your fingers are inside her, gently stimulate this area by tracing around and over her cervix. Then you can combine soft massage with more vigorous thrusting in and out of her vagina while twisting at the wrist so the excitement builds, as she's never quite sure what you're going to do next.

Doing It Her Way

Women masturbate as much as men (even though they don't talk about it) so, just like men, they're the experts on how they like to be touched. A good way to learn about pleasing your partner, therefore, is to rest your fingers on hers while she masturbates herself. Then do the reverse, with her fingers guiding yours. Finally, go it alone, using what you've learned.

The Voodoo Nectars

In one of the first exercises in this book, you met the Sisterhood of the Miracles of Night and were given a magical nectar to drink as part of your initiation into goddess energy (a sweet, honey-based liquid). It is one of the secrets of Voodoo that the body also produces nectars: powerful fluids that are associated with sexual activity and often with the erogenous zones, and that are, in any case, the essence of our sexual powers. Men have five naturally occurring nectars; women have six.

The five nectars that men and women share are sweat, tears, saliva, urine, and sexual fluids (men: sperm; women: vaginal juices). The sixth, which is found only in women, is menstrual blood.

All of these fluids originate in the body and carry our most intimate energies, powers, and personal identity, as well as our DNA. For these reasons, we can use them to produce effects in others. We do so most often in sex magic.

Sweat

Sweat is one of the "clear waters" (*klè dlo*) of the body (the others are tears and, less so, saliva)—the purest emanations of our selves, and, like all waters, associated with emotional energy. By collecting the sweat of your body produced through sexual activity (whether with a partner or alone), you can use it as the basis for a powerful, pheromone-loaded, musky perfume that oozes sex appeal and will bring lovers to you.

A few drops added to a *sant* (see pages 41–44) is all you need, or you can mix your sweat with a blend of two parts patchouli and one part neroli oils and apply it to your pulse points to attract new lovers. Patchouli increases love and passion, and it enhances the satisfaction of sex as well as drives troubles away and manifests wealth and stamina. Neroli is a "magnetic oil," good for attracting whatever you want most.

By applying some of this nectar to your lover (in either an upfront or more sneaky way), you also mark your territory. Smell works subtly, and our moods are affected by it even when we are not conscious of a particular aroma in the air. Your unique aroma will become a *part* of your lover so other potential suitors will know that he or she is yours, and it's "hands off" for them, even if they don't know why!

Tears

Tears are most obviously associated with the emotions—either good (tears of joy) or bad (tears of sorrow)—and can be used in a number of ways.

Tears of joy are used in perfumes like the ones above, or, charged beneath moonlight, they can be used in their pure form to create happiness in others. Applied to a lover's skin, for example, they carry your essence and ensure that he or she is always happy to see you.

Adding a well-chosen spirit-herb or two to the mix enhances the brew and creates other positive effects, depending on what you're after. Pineapple, for example, is used in spells to ensure loyalty, so your lover will only ever want to have sex with you; orange brings love and, if it's what you want, proposals of marriage.

Tears of sadness, appropriately charged with intention, can be used to bring unhappiness to others, such as a love rival or someone you want to punish. Dilute them in dirty water (from a toilet or a ditch, for example) and add three bay leaves (for hexing), then sprinkle this fluid on your rival's doorstep so she is miserable every time she steps over it.

Saliva

Saliva is almost, but not quite, a clear water of the body. Because the mouth is what we use to eat and drink with, our natural fluids are often contaminated with other flavors and additives. To make it *klè dlo*, the best thing is to fast, drinking only mineral water before you use saliva in magical spells. You can also detox, and there is information on this in appendix I.

Saliva is a powerful essence that can be used either negatively or positively. One of its negative uses is to summon your anger and vitriol into it so your saliva becomes a carrier for negative energy (we sometimes do actually spit at people when we're angry with them, and there are well-known expressions like "spitting venom" which suggest the power of saliva in hexing), and using it either in this form or by mixing it with the appropriate dark herbs (henbane— also known as devil's eye or stinking nightshade—would be a good choice) and then finding a way to make your rival touch, absorb, or imbibe it.

More positively, and with good feelings attached, saliva can also be used to mark your lover as your territory—and, if you can get hold of some of his saliva, to mark you as his one-and-only too. Use it as the base for a perfume, and every time he smells it on your skin, he will associate himself with you. Actually, he's smelling (and unconsciously drawn to) his own scent, and this is what attracts him. Vanity, vanity, all is vanity!

The saliva of you and your lover together (collected from a passionate kiss during sex, for example) can produce a powerful binding spell to keep you both together. You only need the tiniest amount because in each kiss we exchange energy and DNA (as well as more than five million bacteria—but don't let that put you off).

Dilute your mixed saliva in fresh, pure water (spring rain is good, or bottled spring water) and add flowers such as marigolds (for brightness and uplifting feelings) and rose petals (for love), as well as a stem of honeysuckle or ivy (both plants wind together with others, as you will wind together with him), and add it to a bath you take together. You'll be lovers for a long, long, time—or until you perform an unbinding spell!

Urine

In Voodoo, the kidneys (which produce urine) are one of our "seats of power": the source of our body's spiritual energy (known as the *nanm*, or soul). This is similar to the concept in Chinese medicine where *jing* is one of the denser and more important of our vital essences or energies and also collects in the kidneys. Urine therefore contains a life force that is uniquely ours. Because of this, it is the perfect substance through which to "stake your claim" or make something (or someone) your own.

Urine also has a scent that is unique to each individual species and to each person. The urine of some carnivores, such as mountain lions and wolves, is even available to buy as a garden aid and will repel pests such as rabbits and squirrels because they recognize through the scent that this is a protected territory belonging to one of their predators.

For related reasons of marking territory and because of the unique energy it carries, urine is often used as an aphrodosiac or during sex magic ceremonies. If you're brave enough to try this for yourself, you and your lover will want to follow a detox diet (see appendix I) for a week or so prior to your ceremony in order to clean out your system, then, for a day in advance of your ritual, drink only fresh, pure water.

Using your first and purest urine of the morning, decant it into separate his and hers glasses, and add honey and rum (warm spiced wine also works well); then retire to your temple, which you will have prepared previously to make as welcoming and exotic as possible, with incense and candles to create a sensual aroma and glow.

Sit on the floor facing each other, a red candle (masculine: for Ogoun and for power) at your side and a pink candle (feminine: for Erzulie and for love) at his, and a white candle between you to signify the union of male and female, you and your lover.

Offer him your glass and say:

I am yours, and I open my gateway to you

After he has taken three sips, he places your glass next to the white candle, picks up his glass, and offers his glass to you as he says:

I travel through your gateway to worlds of love and freedom

Take three sips from his glass, then place it next to the white candle as well. Now pour the remaining liquid into a third glass, so your essences are combined. He offers this to you first and says:

I offer you my power; I offer you my love

Take one sip (enough to drain half the remaining liquid) and say:

I accept your gifts of power and love

Then offer the glass to him, saying:

I offer you my love; I offer you my power

Then he drains the glass and says:

I accept your gifts of love and power

Blow out the white candle and, without getting up, hug each other and kiss.

It is a lovely idea to bring a feast for yourself into the temple to enjoy when this ritual is over. Feeding each other grapes, nectarines, figs, sweetmeats, and other juicy and sexy treats is a beautiful way to celebrate your affection for each other (especially if you've drunk only water the day before)—and then fall into bed for some luscious, unhurried sex!

Sexual Fluids

Sperm and vaginal juices are the quintessential nectars of sexual energy and creation. Like alchemy, their blending gives birth to a third force and, used together, they are the essence of bonding and union.

It is said in Voodoo that sperm is conscious energy; it "knows" its perfect mate and seeks her (or him) out. Sperm is a hunter, a traveler, and, if you think about it, relatively speaking, every sperm crosses a vast ocean in the vagina, driven by an innate and passionate desire to find and fertilize an egg. Men can therefore use the power of sperm in "sneaky magic" to hook a woman (who has an innate desire for her eggs to be fertilized), and it is said that if you can get a woman to unknowingly drink your sperm, she will be yours forever.

The key word, however, is *unknowingly*. During oral sex a woman may swallow, but that is *her* choice and an exercise of her will. Sperm magic works when she drinks in *your* will. So send her chocolates with an interesting center, or make her a romantic dinner for two one night; get the idea?

Now, before women get up in arms about this, the same deal goes for you, except, as a woman, you are the receptive partner, so your magic must be more sneaky still. Use the technique above to draw a lover to you by introducing your essence (by which I mean your vaginal fluids) to something he eats, and he will fall hopelessly in love or lust with you too.

Menstrual Blood

If you loved (or hated) the last technique, you'll love (or hate) this bit of magic even more.

In Voodoo, the vagina (as I said earlier) is the gateway to other dimensions—and menstrual blood is the force that draws in or exudes spirit.

If you are pregnant, your life-blood goes inwards to feed the child in your womb who will then be born from the spirit world: from nothing to something. Every child is a creative idea *you* once had of bringing a new soul into the world. This soul only becomes a real, 3D, living, breathing, physical, material, bonny, bouncing baby through *your* will and essence. You are the one who creates something real and tangible from something unreal and imagined, and your blood is key to this. Your blood *is* the creative life force that links spirit and matter; it *is* the gateway itself.

If you are not pregnant, then your menstrual blood is released; it goes outwards, offering the same possibilities to the world of things that can be imagined and brought into being.

In short: menstrual blood is the voice of the goddess telling humankind that *all is possible*. It's the most powerful nectar there is. (Don't get *too* excited, though, girls, you're only the *gateway* to the divine, not the divine itself. To *be* divine, you'll have to practice your goddess skills so you're really something special and not just a swing-door—which is why you ought to read on!)

How do you use menstrual blood in magic? The world (and beyond) is your oyster. This is *the* healing nectar, the one that can reveal the divine and bring enlightenment to others. Some Voodoo women have been known to introduce menstrual blood to the food they feed their men. By doing so, they say, their men realize their true natures and their purpose as protectors, travelers, explorers of the infinite—those who (like all shamans) visit other worlds and bring back gifts for their tribe and their families. Or, in plainer terms: if you want a hard-working, loyal, never-go-off-the-rails sort of guy who treats you like a princess and puts the family first, feed him your menstrual blood! You only need do it once, so don't get carried away! (You only need a minute amount of blood 'cuz it's DNA we're after—a drop will do, but it must be menstrual, i.e., lost through the vagina.)

The purpose of nectar magic is, of course—and not to put too fine a point on it—to get him into bed and enjoy it when you're there. So the final bit of our basic training is to look at what you do with (and for) him when you get him back to your temple.

Getting to Know You, Part 3:
Sexual Positions

Statistically speaking, every ten times you have sex, two will be so-so, two will be mind-blowing, and six will be good. So look at it this way: every time you have okay-but-no-cigar sex, there's an 80 percent chance that it will get better and a 20 percent chance that you won't stop shaking or sit up straight for days—which gives a whole new meaning to the expression "if at first you don't succeed …"!

There are literally hundreds of sexual positions, each of which creates its own effects and feelings. Some allow for deeper penetration and more vigorous thrusting, while others stimulate the G-spot, and some are more of a cuddle-up with a little penis-thrusting thrown in for good measure. To get the most out of sex, it's good to know a few of these positions so you can find out what you like and accommodate his preferences too.

It's much, much better to be intimately familiar with a few positions, though, than to have an encyclopedic knowledge and not be very good at any of them. So, on the basis that we're looking for quality rather than quantity, here are some of the world's favorites—and, at the end of this section, one special Voodoo technique which, if you learn it well, means you really don't need to worry too much about positions at all!

Women On Top

When the woman is on top, she takes control. This is good for her, allowing her to express her power and dictate the speed and depth of penetration. It's good for the man too, since he can lay still (more or less) and concentrate on his pleasure, which makes a nice change for most men, who are normally expected to climb on top and take care of business.

Here are five of the most popular woman-on-top positions:

The Cowgirl: Your man lies on his back with both legs extended and relaxes most (but obviously not all) of his body. You climb astride him, legs on either side of his body, with your weight on your knees, so you are sitting on him as he enters you. In this position, you are face-to-face, which means you can kiss and cuddle, and you can control the speed of sex and the depth of penetration. If your man gets carried away and starts to thrust upwards, one teasing trick to keep him tantalized is to move your body ever so slightly away so he never quite penetrates you to the depth he'd like. This shows him who's boss (for a change!) and keeps him hot until you're ready to let him take a bit more control.

The Mile High to Paris: Have you ever tried to have sex on a plane? There's really only one position, but it's a good one and can be adapted for use anywhere. Your partner sits down (in this case on the loo seat) and you sit on top, either facing away from him or facing him with your legs astride his hips (you'll need to keep your feet in contact with the floor at least some of the time in order to move your body up and down). You're in charge. Enjoy!

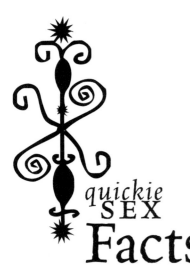

quickie
SEX
Facts!

SEXUAL SHENANIGANS: WOMEN

- 100 percent of women who orgasm can have multiple orgasms; less than 50 percent of them do, though (the most common complaint being lack of clitoral stimulation)
- 85 percent of women need clitoral stimulation to climax
- Stimulating the G-spot leads to ejaculation in 14 percent of women
- 7 percent of women say they fake orgasms almost every time they have sex (girls, you're the ones losing out here, not him!)

The Seesaw: In this position, your partner lies on the bed with his legs outstretched, but with his torso raised, supported by his arms. You climb on top in a mirror-image of his position, with your legs either side of his. You then "see-saw" together, so as he pushes upwards and into you, you lie slightly backwards; then you move forwards as he moves back. As you get the rhythm, you can hold each other and rock forward and backward in that way too. The seesaw gives you limited penetration, so most couples roll on their sides or into one of the other positions for deeper thrusting as their passion increases.

TIM (The Inverted Missionary): In the standard missionary position, the man will be on top, legs fairly straight, and the woman will be on her back beneath him, with her legs more or less straight as well, or else wrapped around her lover. With TIM, the woman's on top, but the position's about the same, and it means he's in the right place for kissing—not only the lips, but the breasts and neck—so you can play around and have fun! Again, you'll probably want to move when things hot up so sex can become more passionate.

The Starfish: Here, he lies flat on the bed and you lie flat on top of him, but with your back on his stomach, so you're facing away from each other. Although you're on top, you don't have much leverage in this position, so movement is mostly up to him and you're in a passive, taking-it-easy role, so close your eyes and luxuriate in the sensations. To add to these, your arms are stretched out to the sides (like a starfish, hence the name), so he has unlimited access to your breasts, nipples, and clitoris for a full-body sexual experience!

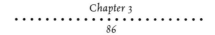
Voodoo Sex Tip: Some women can orgasm through nipple stimulation alone. To increase the sensitivity of yours, massage them for fifteen minutes or so each day with a pinch of cayenne pepper in ginger aromatherapy oil. Then wash off the oil and rub them with juice of aloe vera.

Men On Top

The old ones are often the best—by which I mean men have been on top during sex since the discovery of sex itself, and for very good reason. Forget the women's libbers who tell you that a man on top represents a "negative power relation" and means you don't value yourself; if they actually *had* sex, they'd realize that when he's on top, he's doing all the work—and they can lie back, close their eyes, and enjoy! What's negative about that? When I feel valued, it's often because someone's doing something for me—like giving me an orgasm I don't have to work for!

The important thing is to communicate. He'll be on top, otherwise, thrusting away and thinking he's doing the best for you both, but all he has to go by are his own sensations. Tell your man what you want, or at least make the appropriate noises when he hits the right spot, so he gets the message that way. Then it's a win-win situation.

Here are the classic five men-on-top positions:

The Missionary: He's on top with his legs fairly straight, while you're on your back beneath him. In granny's days (to listen to her speak, anyway), the woman probably kept her legs straight too, didn't move at all, and prayed for salvation as she clutched at her nightie. In these more enlightened times, you'll probably want to bend your legs so you can push your hips up to meet him, or wrap your legs round him so you can pull him into you. This increases the sensation and gives you a bit more control.

The Deck Chair: This one is similar to the Missionary, except your legs are bent and resting on his hips. His are bent, too, so he carries his weight on his knees. This lets him get more power behind his thrusts and means that you can use your calves and your heels to pull him in, raising your hips as you do so, for greater penetration.

The Drill-Down: Lay on your back and raise your legs, bending them at the knees and wrapping them around his back so your calves are resting on his buttocks. He can then scoot forwards so his knees are pressing against your buttocks and his body is over yours, supported by his elbows, which are at the sides of your head. This lets him get a much deeper penetration so you can feel him knocking on the door of your cervix and are completely filled.

Side-on Sex: Lie on your side and raise one of your legs. Your man then positions himself between your legs, kneeling up. By lowering himself so his body is behind you, it becomes almost like spooning. This is a position for playful and unhurried sex, but not one for deep, thrusting passion.

Rear Entry: This is a favorite for women because it allows for deeper pene-tration and, for those who are a little shy or have accidentally gone to bed with a monster, it's great because it means you don't have to look at his face but can bury your head in a pillow instead. You kneel down, with your hips raised high-er than your shoulders, and with your upper body supported by your forearms and elbows, presenting a perfect target to your lover. He kneels behind you, aims for the bullseye and, when he hits it, pushes his hips backwards and for-wards to achieve penetration. By using your forearms for leverage, you can push back to meet his thrusts.

Voodoo Sex Tip: To increase the sensitivity in their penises, Haitian men massage their members for fifteen minutes or so each day with sesame oil. This is said to overcome physical weakness and to help prevent genital and urinary infections. An alternative is avocado, which is thought to increase lust.

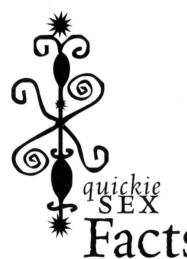

SEXUAL SHENANIGANS: MEN

- The average man ejaculates 5,000 times in his life
- The average length he can "shoot" is 7 to 10 inches, but this can reach 3 feet if he hasn't come for 3 or more days (a foot a day!)
- Impotence affects 10 percent of men; on the other hand, 40 percent of men have a problem with coming too soon
- 50 percent of all people—women and men—have faked an orgasm at some point
- 39 percent of men have kept a sexual memento such as their partner's panties (check your drawers, girls!)

quickie
SEX
Facts!

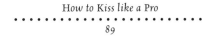
The Infinity Fuck

Sexual positions are great; now you have ten to play with. They allow you to blend with each other, explore yourself and your lover, and find out what turns you on. Knowing your way around a bed and another body means that sex need never be dull.

But sexual gymnastics is only half the fun. As the old adage goes, it's not what you've got but what you do with it that counts—and I promised you at the start of this section a Voodoo technique that makes worrying about positions redundant, because once you know it, it really won't matter what positions you get yourselves into; sex will be mind-blowing in itself.

In Voodoo, it is known that the two great creative forces that joined together to give birth to the universe at the beginning of time are Ayida-Wedo and Damballah, the cosmic serpents whose offspring was the earth and everything on it (including you).

When these serpents are pictured, they're shown as intertwined, curling around each other, and coiling in union. This symbol looks like the snakes of the caduceus, winding around the staff of the healer and magician Asclepius, whose home was the temples where the Horae practiced their magic. It also looks like the double helix of DNA: the code of life that is shared by everyone and everything on earth. The message of the coiled serpents is therefore a simple one: *through sex, all things can be healed.* This single, creative act is fundamental to all life and gives birth to All-That-Is.

Now, if you were to draw a picture of two snakes coiled together, or of DNA strands, and then take a section of it, you'd end up with the infinity symbol, a figure eight, which is also known as the lemniscate:

The infinity symbol stands for life eternal, for the universe as a whole, for the process of death and rebirth, immortality, cosmic exploration, the alpha and omega, and for everything that can be known but is too vast for the human mind to contain. It is one of the most powerful symbols in the universe.

Voodoo has known of this symbol and its use in the creative act of sex for thousands of years, but before now nobody's spoken openly about it or of its use as a method for people to empower themselves through sex. Here's how you use it:

Firstly, get used to the infinity movement. Start by standing up (you don't need a partner for this) and moving your hips. Push them out and to the right, then to the front and to the left, so you complete an arc before you come back to your original standing position. Then do the opposite at the rear: push your hips out to the left, the back, and the right, and come back to your original position. Practice this a few times so you can perform the whole maneuver in one unbroken movement.

Once you've got it, close your eyes and do the same. Visualize yourself taking off as you begin the movement and launching yourself into the cosmos—

the place of the gods and goddesses, home of the *lwa*—then returning safely each time, bringing back wisdom and power which adds more depth and energy to your soul. Keep this up for as long as you wish, or until you feel yourself brimming with power. Now teach your partner how to do it.

To use this creatively in sex, go to your temple together and take off your clothes. Lie on your bed and adopt one of the sexual positions above (the best to try first is the Missionary, simply because it's easier and more straightforward, but it'll work for any position).

When he's inside you, begin to make the infinity movement and keep it up until your movements are synchronized and you are even breathing together. As you push out and to the right, with your eyes closed visualize yourselves launching out of your bodies so your spirits meet each other and mingle above your heads.

See your spirit-selves making love as well, using exactly the same movements, so that their spirits in turn are released, and this process continues until there is a column above you of all your selves making love, with you at the base.

The first couple of times you try this, you probably won't get much beyond three or four couples (or aspects of yourselves) making love in the room, but with practice, this column will grow higher and higher, each of your spirit-selves moving further off into the cosmos to absorb the love and power and wisdom that is found there.

As your lovemaking reaches its climax, or when the feelings in your body dictate, pull your consciousness back into the room and to awareness of your lover and your own pleasure.

You'll experience a wonderful orgasm—but, more than this, you'll return to your body with a new sense of power and understanding.

When your passion subsides and your breathing returns to normal, talk with your partner about all that you've learned. The sharing of experience in this way will always lead to greater intimacy.

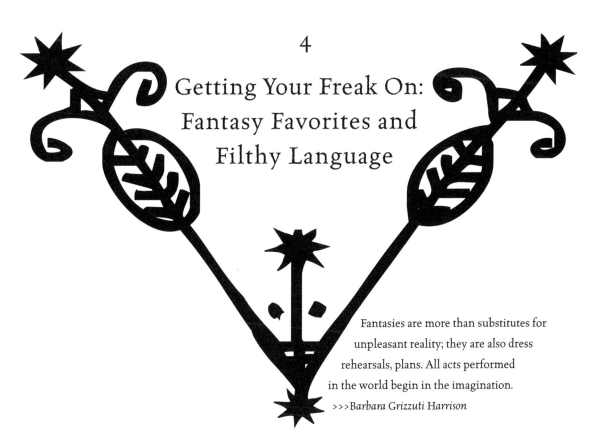

4

Getting Your Freak On: Fantasy Favorites and Filthy Language

Fantasies are more than substitutes for
unpleasant reality; they are also dress
rehearsals, plans. All acts performed
in the world begin in the imagination.
>>>*Barbara Grizzuti Harrison*

In this chapter, we explore freedom-based sex, as opposed to the going-through-the-motions that passes for sex in some people's lives. We look at role-playing, fantasies, and talking dirty: how they spice up your love life and what they have to do with Voodoo.

>>>

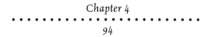
What is "normal" sex, anyway? Is it to do with frequency? And if you have too much of a good thing, are you abnormal?

Well, according to the studies, 33 percent of all men and women have sex, on average, at least twice a week (which means that some must be at it every night), so does that make a third of the population freaks? Unlikely.

The other 66 percent say they have sex a few times a month, a few times a year, or never. On that basis, the most normal thing we can do is not to have sex at all, but clearly we're not doing that or the population wouldn't be exploding the way it is! If frequency is the arbiter of normality, according to this research, anyone who has sex is a freak (I'm proud to be on that list)! So perhaps frequency doesn't tell us very much.

Maybe normality has to do with *who* has sex, then? Perhaps all those young, free singletons are messing things up for the rest of us with their strange, perverted desires? Er, no. Married couples have sex much more often than singles (by a factor of 2:1). And when they're not at it, they're thinking about it: 43 percent of married men and 67 percent of married women (more than men!) think about sex at least once a day.

Well, perhaps it's what you do that makes you nice and normal or a total weirdo? Again, not really. Male-female, penis-vagina sex is the most popular activity for us all, but research shows that people get up to all sorts of things: 75 percent of men and women enjoy oral sex, for example; 20 percent (a fifth of the population) have anal sex; and 57 percent of us buy erotic magazines, films, or sex toys.

As most sex therapists will tell you, in fact—and as those figures seem to prove—there's really no such thing as "normal" sex. Whatever turns you on, works for you, and takes place between two consenting adults is normal—and has nothing to do with anyone else anyway (apart from research companies, it seems)!

What else, according to these kinkily voyeuristic researchers, have you been getting up to in the last year? The 2006 MSNBC Interactive Sex Survey tells me:

- 59 percent of you spiced up your sex lives with naughty lingerie

- 54 percent of you tried new sexual positions

- 40 percent used a vibrator

- 37 percent watched porn together

- 34 percent acted out your sexual fantasies

- 23 percent had anal sex

- 22 percent had sex in public

- 21 percent used food in sex (and it looks like you've got a sweet tooth: chocolate sauce and whipped cream are the things you go for most!)

- 18 percent tried S&M

- 14 percent of you videotaped yourselves having sex

- And 5 percent took part in a threesome

Phew! It's been a busy year! And the more open you were about sex, the better you liked it. The MSNBC survey also asked the question "How long did sex last during your most recent encounter?" The average was 30 minutes when it was dark and there was no sexy talk; 49 minutes when it was dark and there *was* sexy talk; and 53 minutes when the lights were a little brighter and one or both of you were talking dirty!

Given those facts, let's have a look at some of the sexual activities that made the list and see how they relate to Voodoo and our quest for goddess energy.

Mouthing Off

In Voodoo (and in the psychology of body language), to have your head lower than another person's waist is to humble yourself before them and be in service to the spirit—an egoless, open channel for the goddess.

In Haiti, whenever a priest or priestess meets another of higher standing, he or she kneels down in front of them to *dogwe* (kiss the ground at their feet). In the Bible (Luke 7:36–50), we also read that Mary knelt before Jesus and anointed his feet with her tears for the same reason: to be humble.

When we perform oral sex on another, it is also an act of worship. We "give them head" and "go down" before them to recognize their penis or vagina as sacred—a sacrament we take into our mouths. We lose ourselves to another and give ourselves in service so our partners receive not just physical pleasure but, because they are not asked to do anything but enjoy our attentions, they feel loved, honored, and blessed.

Now, here's how to go about it!

Head Skills for Men

Retire to your temple and make sure that the room and your lover are both comfortable. Light some incense and candles and play some appropriately spiritual music (research says that sex lasts longer—and is therefore presumably more fun—when the lights are low and music is playing). Lay your partner on the bed, with a pillow for her hips so her body is slightly raised (this makes things easier for you).

Tell her that what you are about to do for her is an act of worship, to honor her as a goddess—and then describe, in juicy detail, all that you *are* going to do!

(Remember: the research says that sex is better when one or both of you talk "dirty.")

Begin by kissing her, then work your way down her body, licking as you go. When you reach her vagina, use your fingers as well as your mouth: stroke her nipples and vagina while you work your tongue around her clitoris.

Experiment with tongue technique. Vary the pressure, direction, and type of lick: up and down, side to side, circling, using a pointed or soft tongue. Don't forget that she has a G-spot too, which you can stimulate with your fingers. Her reactions will tell you what she likes, so let her writhing and grinding guide you.

Your work doesn't end when she orgasms! Slide up the bed, kissing her body as you go, until you are laying side by side. Hold her and say: "Thank you for letting me honor you," then relax into each other's arms (girls love that sort of thing)!

Voodoo Sex Tip: Try licking her clit with a figure-eight movement, using the infinity symbol described in the last chapter. As you do so, allow yourself to enter a light trance and journey into the "gateway" she offers you, so you draw her goddess energy into you.

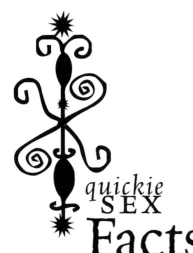

quickie
SEX
Facts!

ORAL TIPS FOR MEN

- 72 percent of women say they prefer up-and-down tongue strokes on the clitoris rather than side-to-side (the figure-eight movement incorporates both)
- It takes an average of 10 minutes for a woman to orgasm through oral sex, so don't give up too quickly!

Head Skills for Women

The oral approach for women is similar: make sure you create a beautiful, relaxing space for your lover, and make him comfortable on the bed. Tell him you want to serve him, and describe how you're going to do it. Kiss his mouth, and slide yourself down his body.

First run your tongue over his testicles, softly sucking each one into your mouth, then lick up the shaft to the glans and circle your tongue around it. You can also use your hands to masturbate him as you suck and lick, varying your rhythm and grip, and cupping and stroking his testicles.

When he orgasms, slide up the bed, kissing him as you go, until you are side by side. Hold him and say, "Thank you for letting me honor you."

Voodoo Sex Tip: Lick him with a figure-eight movement too, up and down the shaft. As you do so, let yourself enter a dreamy, trancelike space and journey into the connective force the penis represents, so you experience the energy of creation.

ORAL TIPS FOR WOMEN

- Oral sex good is for you: semen contains vitamins, protein, and sugars, so it's food for the body as well as the soul
- Every ejaculation contains up to 40 calories—so remember to include oral sex in your diet plans
- Men really like oral sex: 72 percent of them said they even like to get it when they're driving (not the safest option, mind you)
- And it's not just men who like to be in the driving seat: 57 percent of women have also enjoyed oral sex on the road (I've no idea how that works …)

Bottoms Up!

Some research shows that 40 percent of people in the UK and 53 percent in America have tried anal sex. This includes men as well as women, 28 percent of whom have enjoyed anal stimulation from their partners. But before you go poking around in your partner's backside without permission, there are some things you should definitely know, because there's an art to anal play.

Firstly, make sure your partner is okay with it. Some people aren't, and even though 53 percent is a reasonable figure, it still means that 47 percent of the population hasn't yet tried anal sex, so it needs to be something you agree on and not something to plunge straight into!

If you're both happy to proceed, take things slowly. If he's doing it to you, ask your partner to use plenty of lubricant—*on his finger.* Using the finger is the best way to start before he brings out the big gun. Encourage him to make little tickling circles around your anus with his middle finger before he inserts it and, once in, to pay attention to your reactions before he speeds up or changes the pressure.

When you're ready to try the penis, take it slowly and gently again, and use plenty of lubrication. The best position for this, especially if it's your first time, is with you on top in the Cowgirl so you can control the pace and depth of penetration.

Once in, do nothing (or very little) for a few seconds to allow your muscles to relax and so you can get used to it. (It takes some relaxation to accept something as large as a penis in your rectum, and you must feel safe with your lover. If he doesn't believe you, ask him to try shoving a cucumber up his butt and see how he likes it!) When you're ready, your lover should slowly begin to move his penis in and out, only speeding up when you signal that it's okay.

The Power of Sexual Fantasy

More than a third of all people have acted out their sexual fantasies, according to research. But that's not the full story, because a further 22 percent have enjoyed sex in public, 21 percent have used food in sex, 18 percent have tried S&M, 14 percent have videotaped themselves, and 5 percent have enjoyed a threesome. All of these are fantasy scenarios that have been acted out, and if you add all of those figures up it comes to 115 percent—so some of you have been very busy indeed, to a mathematically improbable extent!

Fantasy sex is a powerful thing—especially for women. The Kinsey Institute found that 6.4 percent of women (but only three men in every 5,000) can orgasm by fantasy alone. And yet a lot of people (22 percent of us, actually) are too scared to reveal our fantasies to our partners. Sounds bizarre, doesn't it? We're happy to get naked together and do some of the most intimate things imaginable with videotape and bananas, but ask us to say what we're thinking and we turn into characters from a Jane Austen novel.

But if you won't talk about it, I will, because that's what I'm here for! Your top five fantasies are:

1. Sex with someone of your own gender

2. Sex with a stranger

3. Domination and submission

4. Voyeurism and exhibitionism

5. Group sex and threesomes

Speaking to your partner about your fantasies is liberating and allows a deeper sense of understanding to emerge between you. In *Va-Va-Voodoo*, I gave you the rules for effective relationships: at the top of the list was open, honest, clear communication. If you don't have this and one or both of you is keeping secrets from the other, then your relationship is based on something less than truth because at least one of you lives in a secret world from which your partner is being excluded. Your relationship will be less satisfying, and you will be less fulfilled.

In Voodoo, speaking out loud about who you are or what you've done (*konfyans* or "confession") is a well-known healing technique. When we leave things unsaid, they build up in the soul, changing our spirit and becoming a weight that we drag around with us. To help clients release this stagnating energy, Voodoo practitioners create a welcoming space and use massage and relaxation techniques to set our clients at ease, then ask them to speak freely about anything that's bothering them. This "talking cure" is a similar approach to that used by modern psychologists.

Quite often when clients speak about the things that worry them, they feel better immediately, before any counseling even begins, because a weight is lifted from their minds. Here's how one client put it:

> It's difficult to explain the effects of confession without sounding like a cliché, but it was very much like a "weight off my chest," or rather a weight off my whole body. My physical strength and energy levels seem higher than before, due to the relief of unburdening my "sins."
>
> I came to terms with things I had done—although nothing illegal or heinous, they were the result of a less moral person (my younger self). I had never come to terms with some of these things, instead preferring to try to atone for them without ever facing up to the reality of the consequences that they had on my own emotional well-being. The act of speaking them aloud made me pay attention to what I had done.
>
> As I worked through the emotions, feelings, and thoughts behind each of these "sins," I began to realize why they had occurred, and this gave me greater understanding as to why I had done them. It also allowed me to realize that I had "moved on" from the way of life that led to those actions. By releasing the energy that I had been using to berate myself for my past, I was able to free myself.
>
> In the days after my confession, I felt more confident and more at peace with myself. My energy levels have increased, and I feel more "rounded." I realize that carrying the guilt of previous "bad actions" had been slowing my potential, since I was not using as much of myself as I could be.

I now feel a lot stronger and am keen to make peace with any other out-standing problems and to retrieve as much of my soul as possible. It feels a lot better to have more of me here.

Use "confession" and the Voodoo approach to bring up the subject of sexual fantasies with your lover. Have him lie down on his stomach, naked or with his shirt off at least, and use oils to massage his back, working from the small of the back (where our "serpent energy" is stored), up to the shoulders, and along his upper arms, then release and repeat. This movement is relaxing and will put him at ease, but it also stokes his sexual fires by raising his serpent (kundalini) energy and making him more open and receptive to your words.

Good oils to use are magnolia (for compassion and love), marjoram (which is protective and gives confidence), or jasmine (an aphrodisiac and "the oil of rituals").

Keep in contact with his skin as you speak (or ask him to speak) about the things that turn you on. Since he cannot see you and you are looking only at his back, communication can be more open because you don't have to look each other in the eyes.

When we speak about sexual fantasies—the things we repress—what comes up can be interesting. What we *don't* talk about usually relates to something much wider: how we see ourselves. When we reveal something new, who we are and the way our partners view us also changes, which gives our relationship a new, more powerful, and more positive beginning.

Most sexual fantasies, when you start to look at them, also raise some fascinating questions of their own. Let's take our number three bestseller, domination and submission.

Now, domination to most people means something like "the man (usually) gets to tell the woman what to do, and she gets to serve him sexually. Great! More of the same!"

What they don't know, though, is that (a) women generally—and genuinely—like being told what to do (it's a top-five fantasy), (b) both partners are equal in relationships like this, and domination has nothing to do with spousal abuse or control freakery, and (c)—most interestingly of all—the submissive partner is the one who's really in control of the action.

The submissive must *offer* herself (or himself) for D and S activity. No one can *make* her—and if they try, then it's not D and S at all, but bullying or abuse. She will also give her partner "safe words" so she can tell him whether she's happy with what's going on: green ("I'm okay"), amber ("less okay"), and red ("stop") are typical. When the amber command is given, the person "in charge" will slow down or make his actions less intense; when the red command is given, he will stop. So the person really in control is the submissive, because nothing can happen unless she is okay with it. What the dominant does is facilitate a *spiritual* experience for her—he becomes, in effect, a priest of goddess energy.

Most submissives talk of entering a spiritual place through sexual activity, which they call "subspace." This is a sense of the ego disappearing, so they are no longer worried or concerned about who they are, what they look like, or

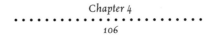
what they habitually do. They are "gone"—an empty channel—and they real-ize that to be in service to another (even though, in reality, they're the ones in control) is the greatest purpose of all.

Subspace, it turns out, is not so different from the Voodoo idea of "posses-sion." When people become possessed during Voodoo ceremonies (called *danse-lwa*), Haitians say that their identity, spirit, or essence goes to Gine (the Voodoo equivalent of heaven) and their bodies are taken over by the *lwa* (the gods and goddesses). In psychology, we'd say that the primary identity (the per-son we think we are) is relaxed so that other potentials and possibilities (the multiple personalities we really are) are given an opportunity to shine. Most psychologists would agree that this is very healing—and that most of us don't do it enough. There's a lot to be said for just letting go!

This is what happens in subspace: people are able to "let go and let God." Instead of suppressing their desires or holding themselves so tight it feels like they're about to burst, they let themselves feel and express.

There is healing information about ourselves in all of our sexual fantasies. You want to have sex with someone of your own gender, for example, or sex with a stranger, or watch your lover with someone else (all top-five fantasies), and that's just the way things are. But if you don't honor that by admitting it (which doesn't mean you have to rush out and *do* it!), there is a part of you that does not fully live.

What's more, all that unexpressed sexual energy is still within you, ferment-ing away—and, as Freud said, if we don't take our unconscious mind by the lapels and look it in the eyes, it bubbles out anyway in actions we didn't intend. It's much better to let this energy flow in situations we can control.

Here's one way of doing it:

Positive Possession

Lay down on your bed and, in your mind's eye, see that inside your body there is a sort of mist that is your essence or *nanm* (soul), which, as you lie there, begins to condense and sink until it becomes a pool that fills maybe only a third of your inner space. In Voodoo, it's said that the soul is like water. When water is heated, its molecules speed up and steam is produced, which fills a bigger space and is hot (fiery, active, passionate); when it cools, it fills less space and is passive. So it is with us: when we are moving, doing things, and need energy, our souls heat up and fill our bodies to give us the life-force for action, but when we lie still and relax, there is more empty space within us, which can be filled with something else—like the power of the *lwa*.

By calling to the spirits you know—Ogoun for power and Erzulie for love—you can fill this space with their energy. State with intent that you want Ogoun to fill you. Then let the rest of you just go to sleep. "Possession" like this, we'd say in psychology, is really a trance where other aspects of ourselves can emerge, so the power that fills us is really our own, which is otherwise usually suppressed.

When you feel a change in yourself, turn to your partner and begin to make love. Feel how it is to be someone else having sex with the man (or woman) you love or lust after—the new ways in which you move, the new sensations you have.

You can play with this state a little as well. Remember: sex with someone of your own gender is a top-five fantasy turn-on, so call the power of Ogoun (or Erzulie) into both of you at the same time, so you're both having sex with vigour, passion, and confidence. Sex with a stranger is also a turn-on—and that's exactly what you're doing here!

Trance states usually last around twenty minutes (just long enough for a lusty romp). After that, take a warm bath with salt and lemon to make sure you're fully back to normal, and drink plenty of water to get your energy moving again. And remember to feed the spirits for their help.

Sex in the Church of Love

While I was thinking about this section of the book, I looked over my notes from a trip to Haiti I took recently so I could attend some Voodoo ceremonies. During one of them, two spirits—Baron and Brigid—took possession of a couple of people there.

Baron is the guardian of the cemetery, the wisdom-keeper and healer you met in my book *Va-Va-Voodoo*, and Brigid is his spirit-wife.

In Voodoo, the spirits have relationships, just as we do. Brigid is regarded as the wife of Baron, but she has an interesting history in her own right. She began as Brid (from whose name we take the word *bride*), the Celtic goddess of love and healing. When Christianity arrived in Ireland, the pagan Brid became the

Catholic Saint Bridgette. The Irish who left to escape the famine took the saint with them to Haiti, where she was recognized as one of the *lwa* and renamed Brigid. She is known today for her healing skills, her creativity, and poetry—talents very similar to Baron's own—which is why, it is said, he married her!

Given a body or two to play around in, these *lwa* get up to some pretty racy sex play and are far from shy about expressing their affection for one another! I thought I'd include my notes here so you can get a feel for what your own lovemaking could be like when you let the spirits move you.

> *The Voodoo priest goes rigid and his eyes begin to roll. The drums quieten for a few beats, then start up again with a new and feverish rhythm. The priest snaps to and begins to dance. Hands on hips, he thrusts his groin toward the drummers and swivels like a Voodoo Elvis, then jerks back as if shot by the drums. He staggers and spins, then charges the drummers as the battle of sound and dance goes on.*
>
> *The congregation understands from these movements that their priest is filled with the spirit and is being "ridden" or "mounted," as Haitians knowingly say, by one of the lwa. Whispers go up from the crowd, and then they cheer as they recognize the spirit by his hip-thrusts: "Baron!"—the guardian of the cemetery and one of the most exciting and best-loved lwa.*
>
> *Barely has Baron been offered his traditional welcome of cigars and rum than a cry goes up from the other end of the peristyle: "Maman Brigid!"*

Brigid, the spirit-wife of Baron, has "entered the head of" (possessed) a woman and begins an equally dirty dance across the dirt to be at her husband's side. The drums are playing wildly now, the people are screaming, the dance is ecstatic.

Baron and Brigid find each other and immediately fall to the ground, sweating and writhing in the middle of the church. When you're suddenly given your life back for a few minutes of a Haitian night, you want to experience it fully! Rum, tobacco, and sex are the things uppermost in your mind (just like any club night)!

The spectacle continues as the mother and father of the dead consummate their marriage before the Voodoo faithful. And then it's over. They come and they go.

The couple stand, looking a bit dazed as the spirits leave them, and they return to their own bodies. They are helped to seats, given water, and slapped on the back by smiling Haitians.

Ladies and gentlemen, Baron and Brigid have left the building—which doesn't mean they won't return at any moment to ride a different body so the dance of life and the goddess continues through them.

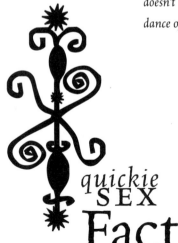

WHAT'S YOUR FANTASY?

- 10 percent of men would like their bottom spanked
- 21 percent of women want to watch their partner have sex with someone else (26 percent of men would like that too!)
- 20 percent of people have used a form of bondage in sex play

Talking Dirty

According to an *Elle*/MSNBC survey, only four in ten people said they'd asked their lovers for a little sexual something in the past month, so a lot of you aren't saying anything in bed—which is a shame because, as I said at the start, sex lasts longer and is more fun when you spice it up with words, and confession is good for the soul.

A lot of sex therapy, in fact, turns out to be education and getting people to talk. A part of my job is teaching people about the power of words—and helping them get their own power back from words that have been used about them.

Take the word *cunt*, for example, which is generally regarded these days as one of the nastiest of sexual swear words. There are various ideas as to where the word came from, one being that it derives from the German *kunton*, which simply means "female genitalia" and is not at all derogatory. Another is that it comes from the Latin word *cunnus*, which means "sheath," although the root of the word also means "to conceal."

All of this is pretty innocent and just demonstrates, if anything, a mysterious, "hidden" power on the part of women. It is only with the rise of Christianity that this everyday word for female genitalia gets a more unpleasant association. By 1230, for example, *cunt* turns up in a London street name: the wonderfully named Gropecunte Lane, which was a street worked by prostitutes. Paris had a street name with the same meaning: *Rue Grattecon*. In both cases, cunt is now associated, not with goddess energy, but with sex for sale, exactly as happened with the Horae. (See chapter 1 for a discussion of Christianity in relation to sexual healing.)

The word *pussy* has a similar history. In the original German, *puse* simply means "vulva," but by the sixteenth century it was used to refer to women in general, a bit like we might call them "babe" or "chick" these days. It wasn't until the nineteenth century that it got a sexual meaning at all, and then, once again, it became a word derogatory toward women (and nowadays toward "effeminate" men as well).

Or take the word *fuck*. According to my friend the Heyeokah Guru, FUCK is an acronym. It originally meant *For Unlawful Carnal Knowledge* and was written on prison doors where prostitutes were locked up for their work as sexual healers.

So, all of these words really stand for *power*—a power that has been taken from women and which will continue to be taken as long as they agree (usually without knowing the origin of these words) that they are in some way "dirty." Women can take back their power when they allow themselves to use words like these as part of their natural and healthy communication with lovers to express who they are and what they want from sex.

Voodoo knows a lot about the power of words. You've probably heard all about "Voodoo curses," where words are used to send energy toward someone and hurt them in some way. But that's really no different to what we all do every day: we get into an argument or express our dislike for someone and, if we're on the receiving end, we know only too well how it feels. That sick, sinking feeling in our stomachs *is* the power of words as negative energy entering our bodies and making us ill.

But words can also be used in healing. In Voodoo, the priestess may chant or sing sacred songs (called *chantes*) over a patient to make him well, or over herbs or special power objects (called *pwen*) to fill them with positive energy. And it's the same with talking "dirty": words can enrich our sex lives, give us freedom, bring us closer to each other, and give us new power. They heal something within us by allowing us to say "Fuck that!" to the shame some people want us to feel about our bodies and our sexual desires.

Here's what I suggest:

- Make a list of all the "dirty" words you've never allowed yourself to use and do some research on their origins. In 99 percent of cases, you'll find that they were all once harmless and innocent and simply referred to parts of the body or to activities that people thought normal.

- Make a commitment to yourself that you'll reclaim your power from these words by facing your fear of using them. Ask yourself where your fear comes from (were you punished as a child for using them, for example, even though you did so in complete innocence?)—and then say "Fuck that!"

- Practice using them (they're only words, after all), saying them out loud to see how they feel. Psychologists call this desensitization:

the more we say (or do) something, the less fearful it becomes and the less of a hold it has on us.

- Then have some fun! Slip a note into your lover's pocket when he goes to work, telling him all the juicy things you want to do to him when he gets home. Here's one I prepared earlier:

  "I want to suck your _____ and _____ you within an inch of your life as soon as you get through the door, you dirty, horny _____"
  (Fill in the blanks to your own taste!)

- Or, if you're normally quiet during sex, allow yourself to make a little noise and let slip with a few choice words next time you make love. Don't forewarn him: just watch the look on his face as you tell him how good his _____ feels!

- And remember: words have a real and physical effect! Sex lasts longer (53 minutes) when one or both of you talks "dirty"—or rather when you're open, honest, and loving enough to really speak your minds!

Channeling Loko and Ayizan
for Cosmic Coupling

Loko Atissou is the patron *lwa* of all *houngans* (priests who work with goddess energy). Once human, Loko was the first priest of Voodoo and did his job so well that he was made a *lwa* himself. He is the "father" of all initiates into Voodoo who come to Haiti to undertake *kanzo* (the special ceremony which creates the priest or priestess) and is represented in the *ounfor* (church) by the *porteau mitan*, the central post, which the *lwa* use like a firefighter's pole to join the congregation.

Loko is also represented as Saint Joseph, Voodoo's father figure, but, interestingly enough, is a *goddess* in African mythology, from where Voodoo comes. He is therefore the masculine (yang) form of goddess energy.

His altar normally features keys (to open the "cosmic doors"), tree branches, herbs, and images of butterflies.

Ayizan Velekete is the "mother" of initiates, the patron of *mambos* (priestesses), and the wife of Loko. She, too, was once human, the first priestess of Voodoo, and became a *lwa* because of her kindness and the power of her work. Images of Christ being baptized by Saint John can be used to represent Ayizan, although her Voodoo symbol is a branch of the royal palm.

Her altar features dirt taken from a crossroads near a market (in Voodoo, the world in which we live is known as "the marketplace" because everything here is for sale—including people—and the crossroads represents the meeting of this world with the next). Her altar might also include water (representing the waters of life and the womb), palms, items bought at a market, plantains, flowers, liqueurs, cane syrup, and yams.

As the first priest and priestess of Voodoo who are both now *lwa*, one of the things that Loko and Ayizan both represent is the importance of communication and union—between the sexes and between the worlds of spirit and matter. Here is a ritual you can use to develop these skills in yourself.

Begin by drawing the *vevers* for Loko (on the left, below) and Ayizan (on the right).

 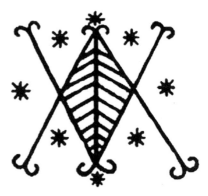

Place these in your temple with a white candle between them, and create altars for these two *lwa* using the items they most prefer: for Loko, keys, herbs, and images of butterflies; for Ayizan, a bowl of water, things from a market, flowers, and a glass of sweet liqueur.

Invoke the *lwa* with the following words:

Loko, who knows spirit

And the spirit of man,

Merge with me and with your wife,

The sacred Ayizan

Bring me your understanding

Of love's true energy

And the importance of connection,

Which flows from the goddess through me

Lay back with your lover and journey, with your drumming tape if you have one, and allow the spirit of these *lwa* to fill you. Meet with them in dreamspace and ask any questions of them you wish about yourself and your part in creation, about your lovers and the roles they have played in your life, and about how you and your sexual partner can work together—physically, emotionally, psychically, and spiritually—to be in tune with each other, and the divine plan for you both.

When you feel you have understood what you need to know about the importance of open communication and the reality of sex as a healing force, open your eyes and come back to normal awareness.

Thank the spirits for their wisdom and clap your hands three times to release them. Blow out the candle.

Then talk with your lover, openly and honestly, about all you have learned and all that love and sex means to you. Tell each other your desires, your needs, your wishes, and your sexy secrets—and then explore these as you enjoy yourselves together!

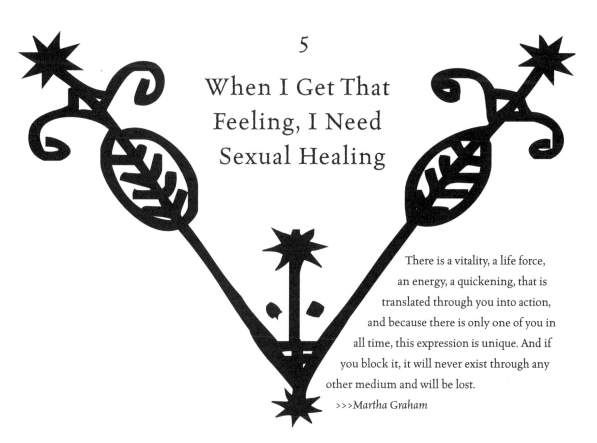

5

When I Get That Feeling, I Need Sexual Healing

There is a vitality, a life force, an energy, a quickening, that is translated through you into action, and because there is only one of you in all time, this expression is unique. And if you block it, it will never exist through any other medium and will be lost.

>>>*Martha Graham*

In this chapter, we get to the nub of what sex is really about in Voodoo. We look at the body's energy system, how sex can empower it and heal us, and how to use serpent flight to open the chakras and become the pythoness: the oracle and seer. It gets a bit technical, but bear with me—it'll be worth it in the end!

>>>

Let's start with probably the most important question of our time: why do men have nipples?

They're no use to them, after all. They're not very exciting as ornaments, you can't milk them, and men don't feed babies, which is what nipples are really about. They do provide a little sexual thrill if you stroke them nicely, but I doubt that's their whole purpose in life, and given a choice between a nipple and an extra penis, I'm sure most men would go for the latter. So what are they doing there?

The answer to that is that for the first six to eight weeks in the womb, all human embryos are female. In plain terms: every person on earth begins life as a woman. Nipples on men are God's way of reminding us that we're all girls inside, and everyone alive is a goddess.

Boys grow out of being female, whereas girls don't. Men therefore experience *two* types of energy: male and female, whereas girls remain girls and grow into women. What this means, in practical (and controversial) terms, is that since all males were once female, they have the potential to understand women better than women understand men. They're also more balanced and can "see both sides" as natural shamans and walkers between worlds, whereas women are just ... well, women (or that's the theory in Voodoo anyway)!

Both sexes, therefore, have access to goddess energy too. It's in us all, so to speak. And in this chapter I'm going to spend a bit of time on that to explain how this energy works and how sex makes it flow, because once the goddess awakes—in a man or in a woman—all sorts of "miracles" are possible.

Goddess Energy in the Body

Firstly, as you probably know, no human being (or anything else) is really made of solid matter. My colleague at the Four Gates Foundation, Ross Heaven, makes this clear in his books when he says that the body's solid bits, if completely compressed, would actually be the size of our thumbs. The rest of us is the space between the atoms, and atoms are held together by energy. Or, to put this in its simplest terms: *we are all energy*. This is what *houngans* and *mambos* mean when they talk about people as having an "energy body" (only they usually call it a soul: *nanm*).

This energy body is not only within us but around us. If you stretch your arms out to your sides, fingertip to fingertip all around you is about the size of your energy body. You know this is true (though you might not know that you know it) because you've probably had that sensation of sensing someone behind you or looking your way, even if you haven't turned around. That's because your energy body is touching theirs, and you're picking up signals from them. (This is also what we do when we flirt with people.)

But there's more to it than that.

This big bubble of energy also has layers to it, and these are your spiritual, emotional, mental, and physical selves. They start at the outside, with the spiritual self furthest away from your physical body. This is where "you" end and infinity—the spiritual universe—begins. Your energy blends with this spiritual universe, and that's *why* you can pick up those signals from the world "out there"—and why you know that Joe Blow fancies you even if he's too shy to buy you a drink.

Your emotional self is a little closer in, a band around eighteen inches thick that begins about twelve inches from your body.

Your mind (or mental) self is the space between your emotional and physical body.

To make this easier to follow, it looks like this:

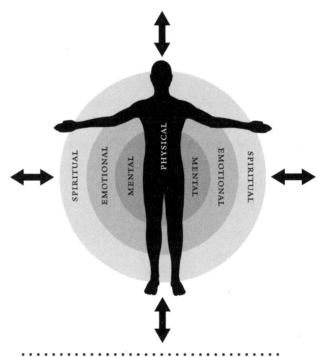

· ·
Your spiritual, emotional, mental, and physical bodies.

The arrows are there to show that there's a two-way flow between *your* energy and that of the world around you. You not only pick up signals (energy emanations) from others, you give them off too.

There is a simple Voodoo test you can apply to see how this energy flow works: sit in the same room as someone you've never met but wouldn't mind getting to know (for example, sit at a table by yourself in a bar). Don't say anything to that person or do anything conspicuous, just concentrate on making him look at you. Send out little threads of energy to tap him on the shoulder and say "Hey!" See if it produces the desired result. If it does, you're in business! And you'll have learned something about Voodoo as well.

Everything that happens to us (or we make happen) in life comes from the world of spirit—or, as we say in the West, the energy of others affects our energy too. In relationship terms, I think it's the same as when some people talk about sensing a chemistry between them: they don't know *why* they feel drawn to a particular person—maybe they're not even their type—but they're drawn to them just the same.

The secret is this: your energy body is in tune with some people and not others, and no matter what your brain or body tell you, your *soul* recognizes the connection between you. At that point, forget it: the little threads of force that surround you both are slowly but surely intertwining to pull you closer together. Depending how in tune you are with the world of spirit, you may even notice it happening.

What happens then is that these energy threads begin to move in toward your physical body, through the emotional layer, and you pick them up as feelings. "Hey! I really like this person!" you say to yourself. "Weird, though—I would never in a million years have gone for him before."

As his little threads continue their journey into your energy, they'll reach your mental self, and then your mind will go to work on the mystery. "Hmmm," you say, "I'd never have fancied him before, but it's his eyes…" (or his suit, or his humor—or the Lamborghini you saw parked outside). Actually, it's none of those things—that's just your mind rationalizing it; it's those little threads of lust and love.

Finally, what began as a spiritual or "chemical" thing ends up with you both in bed. By then, his energy emanations have most definitely reached your physical self!

Because all things work like this and have a spiritual or energetic cause, the Voodoo practitioner has learned to be an expert at manipulating energy, and you can learn it too.

Men *should* be better at this than women, because they began life as females and have goddess energy within them, so they *should* know what women want. This, however (as you well know), is not how it works. Men are rarely that sensitive and, to put not too fine a point on it, if they are, they're probably gay.

The Voodoo answer to this is that knowing too much of their female selves would give men an unfair advantage over women, so the goddess has arranged it so that men's sensitive energies are surrounded by blunter male energy, whereas women are sensitive through and through. The outcome is that men and women can manipulate energy (and each other) equally well.

Try it: visualize sending out a thread of energy from your solar plexus (the place where our willpower is strongest) so it touches another person. Then send out an intention (i.e., a very strong message) to that person along the thread that connects you: "I want you now!" or "Buy me a drink and you might get lucky!" (or anything else you fancy) and watch for their response.

As you get better at this, and if you're with a regular partner, you can also try sitting facing them and sending out the same thread of energy, then transmitting a thought or idea along it. Keep it up for a few minutes to let them get the message, then ask them "What was I thinking?" The couples I counsel find this helps them develop a closeness and deeper rapport with their partner (but don't try it with someone on a first date or they'll probably think you're nuts).

But there's *even more* fun to be had with energy than this!

There are also areas of peak activity within our energy fields, which are known as meridians. Along them are what we call the chakra points (although they're called *sèk limyè*—"circles of light"—in Voodoo, because this is what they look like: small, spiralling wheels of light, which are areas of power on the body). They're most pronounced at the crown, forehead (the "third eye"), throat, heart, solar plexus, perineum, and the soles of the feet. They also connect, in the physical body, to the major organs and important parts of the endocrine system. Working with them to produce energetic effects is therefore like "endocrine alchemy"!

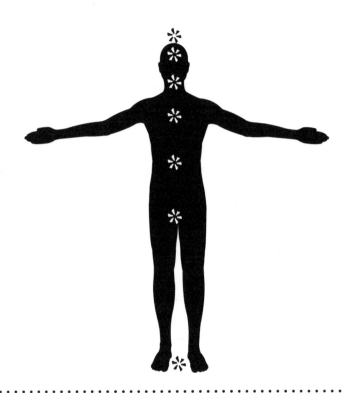

The seven Voodoo chakra points, or sèk limyè; starting at the top: the crown, forehead (the "third eye"), throat, heart, solar plexus, perineum, and the soles of the feet.

You perform this alchemy by focusing on each of your *sèk limyè* in turn and, in your mind's eye, placing one of those little figure eights there (the infinity symbol I talked about earlier). *Sèk limyè* are like the mouths of the energy body, so every time you push this symbol out, you expel energies you've already used from these parts of the body and take in good, clean, powerful energy on the inward thrust of the 8.

Because the *sèk limyè* connect to your endocrine system, this also empowers your physical body and the nectars it produces, making them even more effective in the magic I mentioned in chapter 3.

In Voodoo, we work with the *sèk limyè* to charge them up and produce particular magical effects. For example, if we wanted to attract the man of our dreams (or get a better job, or a new car, or whatever), we'd work on the third eye—for focus—by placing the infinity symbol there. If we wanted more love in our lives, we'd work on the heart. If we wanted more sexual energy, we'd work on the perineum. There is more information on what the other chakras do in my book *Va-Va-Voodoo*, but you catch my drift.

Precisely how we work with the *sèk limyè* is a secret of Voodoo, but I guess I can tell you—and it's to do with another secret: thunderstones!

Thunderstones for Magical Power

There are legends in all cultures of gods and goddesses who cast thunderbolts (power) and lightning (enlightenment) down to earth. This energy was absorbed by the landscape and gave magical potency to its rocks and stones. The stones became the energy of the goddess herself.

Stones like these are known by many different names: *zare mora, sastun,* and *shiva-lingham* are some of them. In Haiti, they're called thunderstones and are revered for their powers.

The Sisterhood of the Miracles of Night teach that thunderstones were formed during the creation of the universe when Damballah and Ayida-Wedo, the snake gods, had sex together and gave birth to all life. In the ecstasy of creation, sparks of magic and nectars (semen and sexual fluids) fell as lightning to the earth. This energy imbedded itself in the landscape, producing natural places of power. Thunderstones contain the essence or soul of this great creative event, and all human beings who touch or walk on them feel the massive energy of cosmic-scale sex.

Thunderstones fell all over the world, and as people walked upon them, sexual rituals were communicated to them through their possession by ravenous deities. The hunger of these deities could only be quelled by offerings of semen, and so women taught men to have sex, and that is how the world's population came to be.

Thunderstones can be found everywhere. Any stone that looks unusual or out of place, has a strange shape to it, or calls you in some way could be a thunderstone. You'll know when you pick one up because it will have a charge to it—an energy you can feel.

Another sign of a thunderstone is that they're often marked with snakelike squiggles, which could be patterns in the rock or natural indentations. This is the mark of Ayida-Wedo and Damballah, the snake gods whose nectars flow in the rock. Those with a mark like this are the most powerful in Voodoo and are used in healing rituals.

If you find a stone like this, hold it in your left hand and blow your intention into it by holding on strongly to an idea of how this stone will help you, then using the breath to blow your thoughts into the rock. This tells the stone what you want from it and wakes up its spirit. This blowing ritual is called a *soplada,* and the stone is held in the left hand because energy flows in a clockwise direction around our energy bodies. When we hold the stone in our left hands, we push our energy into it.

I sometimes collect thunderstones for my clients and have found them in power places worldwide, including Holy Island, Stonehenge, Glastonbury, Haiti, Peru, Greece, and the landscapes around Uluru (Ayers Rock) in Australia. They all have to be collected in a respectful way, of course, ensuring no damage is caused to the environment or to sacred landmarks. I carry out the *soplada* ritual while I focus on my client's needs, then I feed the spirit of the stone by bathing it in a mixture of rum and Florida water.

I like to decorate my thunderstones with original artwork as well, using Voodoo symbols of power to reflect my client's needs. The symbols and the colors I use call other helpful spirits into the stone. When this is done, the stone transforms itself and *becomes* these spirits.

You could decorate your thunderstone with some of the *vevers* in this book or those in *Va-Va-Voodoo*, or with images of snakes: the cosmic and rainbow serpents that embody sexual energy and the qualities of the rainbow—an arc that spans the sky (air), is made from fire and water (raindrops and sun), and connects two places on earth, representing your journey toward power and the treasure that waits at the end of your rainbow. In this way, all of the elements are also called in to serve you.

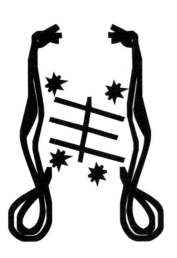

The colors you use will also be significant. In Voodoo, green is the color of Gran Bwa, the *lwa* of healing, which also means peace of mind and harmony of spirit. Red is for Ogoun, the *lwa* of power. White is for purity and also, paradoxically, for sexual power, since it's the color of Damballah, the great serpent sex god! Yellow is bright like the sun and brings balance and soothing to the soul.

Use acrylic paints to decorate your stone and then varnish it so your design will last. Put it on your altar or keep it in your temple when that's done.

Thunderstones are a point of focus for your intention (known in Voodoo as a *pwen*) and will add strength and power to your energy body. You can use them to energize your *sèk limyè* wherever you need their magic by simply lying down and placing the stone on that point. To strengthen your powers of vision, for example, lie down and place the stone on the chakra point of your brow.

Lie quietly for fifteen minutes or so and use the infinity symbol to push your energy into the stone and draw its energy into you. In this way, you create a blending of power and recharge yourself. Be aware of any images or ideas which pop into your mind while you do this, as the spirits communicate through symbols and may give you advice and information as you meditate.

For the same reason, you can also place thunderstones beneath your pillow to enhance your dreaming, or carry them as talismans. If you spend time with your stone—hold it, meditate on it, or journey into it—you may also find other ways to use it as a message from Spirit itself.

Keep your thunderstone fed and charged by placing it outside, on the earth, every three months and leaving it there for one full day (so it is regenerated by the sun) and one full night (so it is infused with gentler moon energy; the time of the full moon is best).

If you read my first book and know how to make *pusanga* (love medicine), it certainly doesn't hurt to rub your stone with a little of this too as it will give you added powers of attraction, so you draw in the good things you want through the gateway of your stone. If you haven't read *Va-Va-Voodoo*, use a scented, sensual oil instead, like magnolia or jasmine for love and prophetic dreams.

Boosting Your Energy Through Sexual Healing

In Voodoo, we know what a healthy energy body looks like. It's a sort of egg-shaped aura around a person, like the egg of the cosmic serpent, slightly wider at the middle than at the head and feet. Its energy spins clockwise, and all the chakras, or *sèk limyè*, are nice and open and flowing. When an energy body looks like this, it's full of power and ready to rock. If we're talking sex here, a partner with an energy body like this can go like a rabbit with Duracell batteries: for hours.

But we also know that it's all too easy for the energy body to get knocked out of whack just by life itself. Sit next to someone on the tube or the bus who's had a lousy day and you're picking up negative energies straightaway. If you've had a bad day yourself, a row with the boss, got it in the neck for forgetting your boyfriend's birthday, or fell foul of anything with an emotional loading to it, your energy body could look like Swiss cheese. More importantly, it'll do one of two things (neither of which is much good for your sex life):

One option is that it'll draw itself into you so it's too close to your physical body. This can happen when we want to make ourselves small and invisible or to hide away from life, or when we're feeling guilty or ashamed. Basically, we're trying to get ourselves out of the way of any flack coming toward us. It can feel like we're under pressure when this happens because energy becomes denser as it occupies a smaller space. We can also get headaches, feel hot, find it harder to breathe, and feel weepy or out-of-sorts. One thing we *don't* feel like is sex!

Another option is that the energy body can "leak" away from us. We get this when we've got a lot on our minds, too many things to do, deadlines to meet, and a thousand different things to take care of—when we're living a modern lifestyle, that is! In this circumstance, we're spreading ourselves too thinly, and this becomes a literal truth as well as a turn of phrase when the energy body responds by spreading *itself* too thinly to try to cope with everything you're doing. This can feel like tiredness, low energy, light-headedness, or a can't-be-bothered feeling—which, in extreme cases, leaves you wandering around like a zombie. Once again, the last thing on your mind is sex!

Which is a shame, because life without sex is … well, life without sex! And a life without a sex life, as Voodoo practitioners know, is a life without spirit, because all things come from sex. Our libido *is* our creative drive, so if you're not making out, you're probably not making anything.

But never fear, because you can help your partner (and yourself) to recover their va-va-voom and get your sex life kicking again with just a little work on the energy body. Here's how you do it.

Chapter 5

You'll Need:

- A pendulum—either shop-bought or homemade by simply attaching a stone, a coin, or a paperclip to a length of thread; and

- Four quartz crystals

And This Is What You Do:

- Have your partner lie down and, although for obvious reasons I'd never suggest this next bit to a client, you can ask him to take off his clothes. There's a reason for doing this in loving (rather than professional) relationships, which is that the effects of what you're about to do will become very visible. Women's breasts and nipples swell by up to 20 percent when they're aroused and their sexual energy is flowing, while men will erect a flag pole, throw a party, and wave you a salute, so you'll know when your healing works!

- Of course, prepare things in advance so the room is warm, there are comfortable rugs to lie on, the lights are low, soothing music is playing, and there's some nice incense burning (sandalwood is great for this).

- Now use a pendulum to show you the shape of your lover's energy body. Hold it over him and work your way out to the four directions of his body. At first the pendulum will probably be still, but it'll start to move when it reaches the boundary of his energy field. In normal circumstances, this will be an arm's length from his physical body, but in situations of stress or other problems, it might only be a few inches away or, alternatively, might look like it's on its way to Outer Mongolia to avoid the problems of being here now!

· When you reach the boundary of your lover's energy, put one of your quartz crystals down on the floor to mark it. Carry on until all the directions are covered. You will be left with an energy map made up of the crystals that now surround him. It will look something like this:

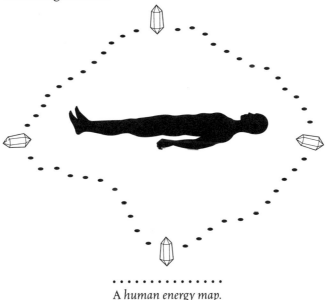

A human energy map.

- If his energy is too far away from where it should be—an arm's length from the body—use your hands to find it (you'll feel a temperature change at the boundary or your hands may shake or tingle), then push it back to where it belongs. If it's too close in, do the opposite and push it away.

- Use the pendulum again to check that it's moved, then reposition the crystals to map the energy body's new position.

- Now hold the pendulum over each *sèk limyè* in turn and see if these are spinning in the right (clockwise) direction. If they are, the pendulum will also spin that way. If it doesn't move, moves to and fro, or spins in the wrong direction, push the palm of your hand into his energy field at the relevant point and around in a clockwise direction, like turning a wheel, to spin his energy back in the right direction. (See illustration on page 126 for *sèk limyè* locations.)

- When you've done all of the above, your lover will have a properly aligned energy body—and a lot more get-up-and-go to demonstrate his thanks for the healing!

There's something else you can do for him to bring his attention back to what's important in life and keep his energy body pumped up with sexual power, and that's to use Voodoo herbal medicine.

When we forget what's important (being alive and enjoying it), we get caught up in all sorts of ridiculous dramas (pleasing the boss, keeping Mom and Dad happy, having the "perfect" figure—you name it!), but what we don't do is *live*! And that's a waste of our time. Medicine—healing—is about bringing us back to what's real so that we conserve our energy and use it for what's worthwhile and good for us. Most of the time (just in case I need to say this again), that's sex and loving relationships!

So here's some medicine you can try. In the West, we call these aphrodisiacs, but in Voodoo they're sexual energies. (Also see appendix 2.)

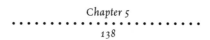
Voodoo Aphrodisiacs

For Him

In Haiti and in the Amazon, the absolute key ingredient of aphrodisiacs for men is bamboo, because bamboo does not bend in the wind, if you see what I mean! An alternative is sugar cane, but bamboo is stronger and better. To give your man sexual energy, you'll need the following:

- A length of strong bamboo or sugar cane (6–9 inches long)

- A teaspoon of ginseng

- A teaspoon of damiana

- A teaspoon of grated *uña de gato* (cat's claw) bark

- A square of natural fabric to wrap the bamboo in

- A glass bottle in which to put these ingredients

- A teaspoon or two of honey

- Rum or vodka

Wrap the bamboo, ginseng, damiana, and cat's claw in natural fabric and bury it six inches below the ground for seven days. Six to seven inches is the length of the average male penis, remember, girls? But if you're looking for a *real* adventure, try burying it nine inches deep for nine days!

After this, dig it up and put all of these ingredients into the bottle along with the honey, and add the vodka or rum (five-star Barbancourt rum is traditional in Haiti). You can also add any nectars you wish (see chapter 3), if you want to create particular effects, like loyalty in your man.

Then make an altar for Ogoun and Erzulie. This need only be a plate of food for each of them, with a red candle for Ogoun and a pink one for Erzulie, and a white candle between the plates for you. Put the bottle between the plates and light the candles.

Then say:

> *Erzulie, this is for you;*
> *Feed and sustain my man!*
> *Ogoun, this is for you;*
> *Bring him the power to stand!*

Leave the bottle there until the candles burn down and the spirits are fed, by which time they'll have heard your petition. Then you can use the brew as a tonic.

If your man is down with the program and knows what this medicine is for, he can take a tablespoon or so of the brew each morning and night to get his juices flowing. If you're using sneaky magic—or if he's *very* down with the program—he can drink it any time he likes (it's delicious) and especially before any important business you have to take care of together.

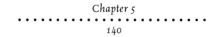
For Her

The key ingredient in aphrodisiacs for women is passion fruit. Other soft, moist, sensual fruits like kiwi or pomegranate are okay too, but passion fruit is the love medicine *par excellence*—even its name tells you so!

To give another woman—or yourself—more sexual energy, you'll need:

- The pulp of a whole passion fruit, sieved so the juice can be used without the bits

- 3 hibiscus flowers

- A teaspoon of cinnamon

- A teaspoon of ginseng

- A half-teaspoon of coriander

- Rum or vodka

- A teaspoon of honey

- A glass bottle in which to put the ingredients

Mix it all together in the bottle (along with any nectars you wish to add), cover the herbs with the vodka or rum, and float the hibiscus flowers on top. Place the bottle in direct sunlight for one hour at midday for three consecutive days. This fills the mixture with power and, since the sun is a masculine energy, it'll also help you cut through sexual inhibitions (something men are better at than women, because they've *been* women at one stage but overcome their female hang-ups through male energy).

When this is done, create an altar in exactly the same way as above. Put the bottle between the plates and light the candles. Then say:

Ogoun, this is for you;
Release my/her sexual power!
Erzulie, this is for you,
So my/her sexual strength may flower!

Leave the bottle there until the candles burn down, then you can use the brew. Take a tablespoon morning and night or drink it at any time (a couple of glasses never hurt!)—and especially before he whisks you off in his strong arms to bed (with your consent, of course)!

THE STUFF THAT GETS YOU GOING!

The top 10 aphrodisiacs (in order) are:

- Oysters
- Truffles
- Chocolate (yippee!)
- Caviar
- Cheese (huh?)
- Bananas
- Pomegranate
- Ginger
- Chili (just don't overdo it!), and
- Ginseng

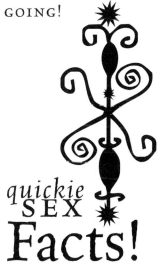

quickie SEX Facts!

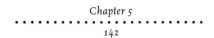

The Pythoness Sexual Oracle

I said at the beginning of this chapter that sexual energy, flowing in a good way, makes all sorts of miracles possible. Of course, they're not really miracles since everyone's capable of the miraculous when their healthy, creative juices are flowing. When your energy system's in balance, it's in contact with the energy of the universe, and there's a healthy connection between you and everything else. One way that the Sisters of the Miracles of Night use this is to become the pythoness: the oracle or seer.

According to the sisterhood, above the doorway to the temples of Aphrodite there used to be a sign: *Know Yourself*. It was the work of the sacred slut to reveal this truth to their clients: that their real life's mission was to know who they were. This knowledge would lead to love and happiness because the ultimate truth we all have to learn is that *everything* in the universe is love. This is the energy that makes all things possible. When people understand this and live in love, there is no room for conflict in the world; when everyone is happy and their needs are met, there are no more disappointments that lead to want and to war.

Knowing yourself (and others) for who you/they truly are is vital to your spiritual well-being. And life is short! To make the most of it, you ought to know, for example, if the man you're with is really going to make you happy; if, through him, you're going to find satisfaction, if you're ever going to get the Lamborghini, or if you should cut and run. Then you won't be wasting the precious time you have.

Want to know how it's done—how to become a pythoness, so you can ask questions of the spirits and find answers that make you happy? This is how it works:

- Firstly, you absolutely must be in touch with your sexual energy. Visualize a coiled serpent in the small of your back, just above your buttocks, and see it unwinding and beginning a journey up your spine, over your head, and into your third eye. When it gets there, you are serpent energy: the pythoness.

- You absolutely must use incense. The oracles of Delphi and the priestesses of Aphrodite burned herbs to take them into altered states. In Haiti, the aroma of Florida water, a heady and aromatic perfume, is most often used, but if you can't get hold of this (there's a recipe for it in *Va-Va-Voodoo*), one easily found incense you can use, which has long been popular in rituals of this kind, is frankincense. Light it, sit in its smoke, and breathe it in.

- You absolutely must be in darkness. Sit in a darkened room or place a shawl or blanket over your head. In Voodoo, pythoness divinations are conducted in the *djevo*, the dark inner sanctum of the temple. The oracles of Delphi sat in caves and hid their faces beneath sheets to shut out the world. Either method is fine. Then close your eyes and, through a combination of sexual energy— the serpent flight rising up your spine and the aroma surrounding you—reality will start to shift, giving entrance to the world of spirit.

- Ask any questions you like: "How do I find a new lover?" "How do I keep him true?" "How do I let myself go further sexually—what's stopping me?" Or anything else you want to know.

- Speak your answers out loud, as the oracles do. It may be useful to have a tape recorder, but if not, just keep talking in a stream of consciousness until you feel like stopping. Then write down what you remember.

- One question you can always ask is "How can I serve the goddess by becoming a better lover and sexual healer?" Knowing the answer to that could tell you the most important thing of all: your true purpose in life.

Dirty Dancing

In Voodoo, dance is used to get into the energy body and out of the conditioned mind. Dancers "sweat their prayers," as Gabrielle Roth puts it, so they lose themselves and the spirit enters them. Power fills them as serpent energy uncoils in their bodies.

The music they dance to is the drums. Every rhythm the drummers play is a call to a particular *lwa*, each of which has their own drum signatures and particular style of dancing.

Gran Bwa is the spirit of nature, and when his energy courses through you, you will develop an intuitive knowledge of plants and their use in magic. His dancing has the power of the trees, and his steps are "rooted" and strong.

Erzulie moves in a stylized way, sometimes floating and gliding like a ballerina or at others like a vamp who wants to dance with as many men as she can.

Ogoun, because he stands for power in all forms, can move with the refined air and grace of a diplomat dancing at a lavish ball or with the wild, energetic leaps of a young warrior at a tribal fire, expressing his lust and strength.

My personal favorite is Baron, who's really quite a mover, and whose dancing is a celebration of life! He has his own bawdy dance called the *banda*, which is full of pelvic thrusts and explicit hip movements. He is a "phallic" *lwa*, says Laennec Hurbon, a Haitian professor who writes about Voodoo. All of the *gedes* (the family of the dead, of which Baron is the father) "tell dirty stories, perform lascivious and obscene dances, and spend their time playing jokes on the Voodoo faithful … The eccentric behaviour of [Baron] expresses the art of turning death into satire. Playing death in order to outwit it—this may be [his] scheme, for if death is unavoidable, outplaying it with life lets one face it successfully."

Dancing and drumming, as Voodoo practitioners know, carry the spirit of healing within them. Science is catching up with this too. Research into stress, for example, shows that one of the problems of modern life is that we are under constant pressure as a result of our way of living. Our energy gets stirred up to deal with stressful events but is hardly ever released, so it accumulates in our systems.

One of the solutions scientists have found is body movement and dance, which lets us use our stuck energy in a way that is helpful, leading to lower levels of depression and hypertension, and reductions in heart rate and blood pressure. We relax, let go, and move closer to Spirit when we dance. Or, as Gabrielle Roth puts it, "The more you dance, the more you sweat. The more you sweat, the more you pray. The more you pray, the closer you come to ecstasy."

Drumming has the same effect. It changes our brain waves to a more calming theta range, which is associated with relaxation, dreaming, and trance, and is good for us in all sorts of ways.

So, when we dance or drum, healing takes place on three levels: we reduce the effects of stress by freeing our pent-up energies, shifting our brain waves, and releasing feel-good endorphins into our bloodstreams; our imagination and its intuitive powers are stimulated; and the spirits can enter us to offer their healing too.

If you want to dance with the *lwa* and get your own sexual powers flowing, try the *banda*. Stand with your legs slightly apart, hands on hips, and rotate your hips in the figure-eight infinity movement I talked about earlier. Keep this up for five to ten minutes and it'll lull you into a light trance. Call to the spirits at that point, and ask them to reveal their healing and sexual secrets.

The *banda* is a dance of how low you can go and proceeds by opening the legs wider and wider while keeping up the hip rotations. If you're stretchy enough, you'll end up in a full split—or at least you'll be close enough to the ground to simply flop down and journey in the way I've described before, so you can meet the spirits and speak with them. At the same time, a delicious, warm glow will be spreading throughout your loins as a result of all your dancing. Bliss!

When our energies are flowing and we feel good in ourselves, dancing almost always leads to sex! If you're in a nightclub at the time, it may not be a simple hop, skip, and a jump from the dance floor to the boudoir, but a jump is usually involved in it somewhere. Dancing leads to touch and then to kissing in every courtship ritual. That's how it is with flirting: it moves from the floor, to a drink, to a chat, a light caress, and a kiss—and it's up to you where it ends.

Never, ever underestimate the erotic power of dance to convey sexual healing—or to get a man to do your bidding! Even the Bible's clear on this. The Gospel of Mark tells the story of Salomé, the infamous dancer of the seven veils, and her ability to twist any man around her finger.

In this story, Salomé's mother, Herodias, has an adulterous affair with Herod, and both of them leave their spouses so they can marry. John the Baptist didn't much like this and spoke out against it. Herod had him imprisoned for this but not killed, despite Herodias's wishes (the female of the species being deadlier than the male and all).

Herodias had a secret weapon for getting her own way, though: her daughter Salomé. During a celebration for Herod's birthday, Herodias had her sexy young daughter dance for Herod and his guests, who each peeled off a layer of her clothes—seven veils in all—until she was wearing next to nothing.

Herod was so turned on that he made an oath right there and then that Salomé could have whatever she wanted. "Ask me for anything," he panted, "even half of my kingdom, and I will give it to you!"

Salomé (nice girl!) asked for the head of John the Baptist on a plate. Even though Herod didn't exactly want to go along with this, he had to make good on his oath—and that's how John (and Herod) both lost their heads, according to Mark!

And here's how you can use dirty dancing to get what *you* want from your man:

The Voodoo Striptease!

- Set up your temple and make it lush and inviting. Lighting is important for what you're about to do because you want your man to see and appreciate your body but still leave something to his imagination. Candles and/or side lights are best. Have two chairs in the room as well: one for you and one for him, positioned so you can move around it.

- Sit him in his chair and tell him to relax and enjoy. Then put on some music—something seductive but with a strong, deep bass line: remember the power of the Voodoo drums for sending you both into sexual trance!

- Explain the rules of the game: that he can look but he better not touch! He can face front, turn his head, or look over his shoulder, but his backside must stay on the chair and his hands remain at his sides. You may even want to tie his hands to the chair. He is not allowed to speak either—no questions, interruptions, or requests, thank you—unless you ask him to. Tell him who's in charge, then leave the room for a while and let the sexual tension build!

- While you're gone, it's time for you to quick-change into something sexy. Have it prepared in advance and remember the "tease" in striptease. You want layers of shear, slinky, and clingy clothing— your own version of the seven veils—something you can open easily and give him flashes, then cover up again, to maintain the sexual tension! White is a great color for striptease: there's something really dirty about a pure and virginal color in a hot performance like this. Or wear black and red, the colors of the vamp.

- A few style tips: wear a skirt (short and sexy) or something more sophisticated, like a ballgown. Both are equally good for different reasons, depending on the effect you want to create, but whatever you choose, make sure it has a zipper or buttons, definitely not an elastic waist (too frumpy). Buttons and zippers also give you something to work with. Same with your top: a button-up blouse is great, but not a T-shirt! Wear stockings (not pantyhose), a bra that conceals your nipples (don't give him too much too soon!), and panties with lace and frills, but not a thong (again, don't give everything away at once). Shoes with a heel will make your

stockinged legs go on forever and give you extra poise. Jewelry—
like a necklace that hangs between your breasts—adds to the effect,
and you can play with it suggestively. For the finishing touches, fix
your hair, do your makeup, and apply a little *sant* or even an
ordinary perfume (but something a little racier than normal).

• Enter the room and circle his chair slowly, giving him a good look
  at you. Whisper in his ear, telling him you're going to make him
  soooooo hot—and there's nothing he can do about it! Run your
  fingers over his chest or through his hair as you walk around him.
  Maybe run your hand up his thigh, or straddle one of his legs and
  grind yourself into him.

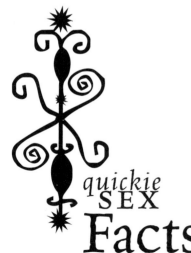

quickie
SEX
Facts!

DRESSING FOR SEX

• **80 percent of men are turned on by sexy lingerie**
• **40 percent of men don't know how to remove a bra;
  teach him!**
• **70 percent of women aren't comfortable undressing in front of
  men—so think of the advantages you'll have and how you'll
  stay in his memory after a sexy striptease like this!**

- Then, just as he's enjoying it, step away! Begin to dance, keeping your moves slow and sensual and your hips in motion. Overemphasize your movements when you walk and turn, like one of those '50s film stars. It's all in the hips, believe me! You'll mostly want to be in front of him, a few feet from where he's sitting, but it's sometimes good to go behind him too and brush against him ever so slightly; it keeps him guessing. Get real close from time to time as well and rub against him with your breasts and groin—but it's always hands-off for him!

- Use your chair: put one leg on it to peel down your stockings; sit on it and slowly part your legs, like Sharon Stone (but with a bit more sophistication, please) in *Basic Instinct*; or bend over the back of it so the tops of your breasts are on show.

- Play with your clothes as you lose them. Keep it slow: one button at a time, a quick peek here, a flash there, covering up and revealing, before you finally take them off. Remember the tease. Play with yourself as well, stroking, squeezing, and rubbing. Men love to watch an uninhibited woman enjoying herself! Heighten the effect by telling him what you're doing and how it feels. "Ooooh, my nipples are so hard!" "I feel so horny!" Use your imagination!

- At the end of your dance, make sure you're still wearing stockings (men love them: they frame the vagina and focus the attention nicely, and they work wonders for your thighs), and keep the jewelry you had on at the start (provided you're not dripping in it) so you have something to twiddle.

• Now that you're naked, grind your hips, forwards and backwards, in a figure eight. This infinity movement, as we know (even if he doesn't), lets you direct sexual energy straight toward your man. Open your legs a little as you continue these movements, showing him more and more of your sexual power and inner self.

• Finish by masturbating in front of him and bringing yourself to orgasm. This will drive him wild, not least because he has to watch but still can't touch!

• Don't get too carried away and completely neglect him, though; the show was for him, after all! You can give him an orgasm in the chair, using your oral skills, or climb on top of him in the Cowgirl or Mile High position—or you could be nice and untie him so he can take you to bed and show you how grateful he is!

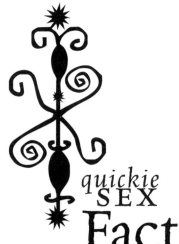

quickie
SEX
Facts!

YOUR TANTRIC ADVANTAGE

• **Only 7 percent of people have used Tantric practices like dirty dancing and striptease in their sex play; think of the advantage you'll have over rivals when you become a goddess of the art!**

Voodoo Sex Toys

Toys are popular in sex, and vibrators are our best-loved playthings: 20 percent of adults say they've used one.

There are some cultural differences, though. Americans and Brits are most likely to own a vibrator (43 percent of us have a little buzzing friend in our bedside cabinets), but it's the Taiwanese who top the chart with 47 percent—almost half the population (presumably the female half!) having one at hand.

Indians are more reserved, though, and 52 percent say they'd never buy such a thing! So it pays to know who you're playing with and their preferences in matters like these before you take an Indian home and scare him half to death when you open your drawer full of sex aids.

If toys are your thing, there are some spiritual tools in Voodoo you can use to make your play more pleasurable—and a healing experience too.

The Chacapa

This is used in the Amazon more than in Haiti. It's a bundle of dried leaves that shamans use to straighten out kinks in the energy body.

As I said earlier, we can pick up energies from others even by just sitting next to them, because our energy bodies mingle. By running a chacapa through your lover's energy body, just above the skin, you can scoop out the imperfections as negative energies attach themselves to the leaves. The chacapa is then shaken to throw off the energies you don't want on him or in you.

Sometimes shamans use a chacapa to lightly beat the skin as well. This is good for the energy and for the physical body, bringing the blood to the surface, helping to release toxins—and it feels wonderful, like a massage! You can, of course, also run the leaves lightly over the erogenous zones for a deliciously horny tickling sensation.

To make a chacapa, you just need to collect some leaves and allow them to dry naturally for a few days, then bind them together with string. They need to be fairly long leaves—the magical six inches or so!—and not too brittle, so they won't crumble when you use them.

Remember that all plants are owned by the *lwa* of the forest, Gran Bwa, so leave a gift for him near the bush you collect them from, and tell him what you'll be using them for. Then he can empower the leaves to help you enjoy them more.

Feathers

Feathers are another energy tool in Haiti. Held delicately and run through the energy field that surrounds us, they're a diagnostic aid to show you where there's a build-up of energy in the body. When the feather reaches a blockage, it will dip toward the skin or sometimes be pushed away as if it were hitting a physical object. If this happens, the shaman will use the tip of the feather like a knife to cut out the negativity and scoop it up. He'll then release it by blowing on the feather to cast it away.

If you try this on your partner, remember that feathers are also soft, gentle, and tickly! There are some lovely, sensitive parts of the body—like the inner thighs, breasts, arms, and torso—where you can use them to delicious effect.

A feather run gently and repeatedly over the clitoris or along the penis can feel very nice indeed!

Clean your feathers after use to make sure there are no negative energies stuck to them. Just hold them in sage smoke for a while and they'll soon be as good as new!

Whips

In Voodoo, whips are used to frighten away bad spirits and to wake up the spirits you *do* want on your side.

On a walk in Haiti to collect magical herbs from the forest, for example, the lead *houngan* will carry a whip, cracking it regularly to keep the spirits at bay. When he reaches the tree he wants to take leaves from, he'll crack the whip again, shouting "*Travail! Travail!*"—"Work! Work!"—so the energy of the tree flows into the leaves and empowers them. Only then will he pick them.

Sometimes whips are used, lightly, on the body of a patient as well, and for the same reasons: to scare off the bad spirits (or energies) that person is carrying and get his good energies flowing again.

If you want to incorporate a whip into your sex play, there's absolutely no need to buy one. A few strips of leather, about nine inches long, can simply be tied together for a cat-o-nine-tails, or you can use a piece of rope, which is what most *houngan's* whips in Haiti are made from.

Always whip your partner lightly unless he tells you he'd like a little more force, and stay away from bony areas like the shoulders and spine, where a whip can really hurt even if you do use it gently. The idea is to make it a sensuous experience and bring a rosy glow to softer and more padded areas, like the buttocks and thighs, not to scar him for life! So choose your targets carefully.

If you want to use it for healing as well, *very gently* whip the stomach, genitals, the top of the buttocks, backs of the knees, and the backs of the elbows by running the thongs over these areas. These "angles and corners" of the body are where bad energies tend to accumulate. Whipping them brings these energies to the surface in the form of heat so they can be removed.

Follow a good whipping with a soothing bath of chamomile and rose petals, or a massage using a few sprigs of mint in a base oil, to cool the body down and release the negative energy completely.

Nettles

This one's not for the faint-hearted!

Nettles are sometimes used in the same way as the whip: to bring energy to the surface. Using them on the skin creates heat and a prickly sensation that draws these energies (or "spirit intrusions," as they're sometimes called in Voodoo) to the skin. At that point, you can use your feather to scoop them away, or take the bath or massage I've already recommended.

Some people like the sensation of being stung and, once they overcome their fear of it, find that it doesn't actually hurt that much. Then, when the feather is run over the stung area, the contrast is exquisite, the skin is so much more sensitive, and they start to relax and get turned on by it. See how you like it, if you're brave enough to try!

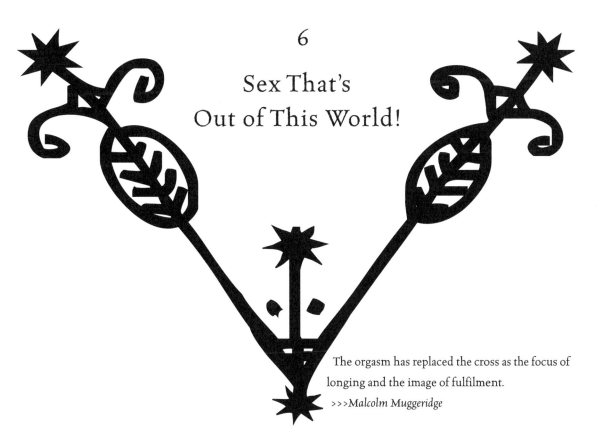

6

Sex That's Out of This World!

The orgasm has replaced the cross as the focus of longing and the image of fulfilment.

>>>*Malcolm Muggeridge*

Now that we've looked at the energy body—what it is and some of the things you can do with it—in this chapter I'm going to talk about more advanced energy techniques: astral projection and astral sex.

Then we're going to come right back down to earth again and learn to appreciate our physical bodies and the gifts of nature. Finally, there's another little initiation for you into goddess energy that takes place in the dark!

>>>

Here's something interesting I read the other day: psychologists at universities in England have discovered that artists and poets have about twice as much sex as us mere mortals. Creativity is like a sexual magnet, and the more creative, open, and intuitive we are, the more sex we get.

The psychologists carried out a survey of 425 British men and women, including artists and poets, and found that the creatives had up to ten sexual partners, while the others had three. The number of sexual partners increased as creative output went up.

History tells us that Picasso, Byron, Dylan Thomas, Richard Burton, and other well-known artists and rakes were at it almost constantly, and that's no coincidence. They were all highly creative and highly sexed. The two go hand in hand.

I've been saying the same thing for years! (Why do these scientists never ask me before they spend a small fortune on surveys?) If you look at any creative culture, like Haiti or the Amazon, they're all more relaxed about sex and more practiced at it than the stuffed shirts and uptight commuters we have to look at on the train every day.

They're also all dreaming cultures: they use imagination, fire, creativity, and passion to get things done, and they talk about energy and spirit. They know the "otherworld" in the same way that artists, poets, actors, and musicians have to know it in order to do their work.

So, in short: the more creative you are, the more sexual you'll be *and* the more sex you'll get. It pays to develop your dream power (as *Reader's Digest* almost used to say), and that's what this chapter's about.

The Dreaming Universe

All dreaming cultures know that we really live in two worlds: the one we see around us and the one we can't always see but is there nonetheless, and is where the spirits, intuition, and creativity come from. In Haiti, this invisible world is called Gine. It's like Voodoo heaven or the Garden of Eden.

When people are possessed in Haiti, the spirits come down from Gine and enter the body so the *lwa* become "human" for a while. At the same time, the spirit of the person possessed goes to Gine, where it's protected and healed by the other *lwa*.

If you ask people what Gine is like when they come back to their bodies, sometimes they remember and describe it as a beautiful forest or a magnificent temple, which sounds a lot like those of the Horae. While they're in this paradise, they're pampered and fussed over and all their wishes are fulfilled. They can go anywhere, do anything, and find they have new powers. Sometimes they visit other places on the planet, past lives, or future possibilities; have sex with strangers, gods, or people they know; and eat delicious foods, drink wine, and listen to beautiful music. It sounds divine. Well, I guess it *is* divine!

Possession, as I've said before, is a trance state—a type of dreaming—where we're relaxed and open to spirit, and the visit to Gine is a form of astral projection. We're so "open," that is, that our spirits can leave our bodies and take us wherever we want to go. To put this in the terms we used last chapter, we detach our energy from our physical selves so we can feel, think, imagine, create, and experience wonders while our bodies remain on earth.

But you don't even need to be possessed to do all of this. *Vòl nanm* (soul flight) or astral projection will get you there too!

Learning to astral project is really quite easy once you understand and accept that you have an energy body and can use it to journey out of your physical self and into the energy realms.

The energy (or astral) body is made of light, which is not held down by gravity or subject to the laws of physics. It can move by thought alone, fly, walk through walls, dive to the bed of the ocean, or visit the stars. It doesn't need food, clothes, or even oxygen, and it can't be hurt or injured. Communication in the astral body is by thought alone (telepathy), so there's no need to move our lips when we speak or use our ears to hear; we simply transmit our thoughts and ideas and pick up on the thoughts of others.

Time and space have no meaning in the astral world either. A single thought will get you from New York to New Delhi in an instant. You can "time-travel" too (since there's no such thing as "time" to begin with), which means you can visit loved ones who have passed on and connect with them again or journey to the "future" to see how things might turn out for you or others (precognition). The ancestors, or *zanset yo*—loved ones who have passed over—by the way, are considered among the most important of spiritual guides in Voodoo. They have been human, so they understand what it's like, the problems we face, and the needs that we have, but now they are spirit and have greater wisdom and power, so they can provide us with loving guidance and sound advice—something to bear in mind for your travels.

All things begin as thoughtforms. You can't make a cake (or a baby, a bomb, or a baseball bat, for that matter) without dreaming it into existence. Because the astral is the "world of ideas" from which all creative thoughts come, it also contains things that you won't see on earth—anything you can imagine, in fact—because they haven't yet been plucked from the ether by the creative people who will turn them into physical things. So expect to see the unusual, the bizarre, and the brilliant, as well as things you recognize! In a sense, you're seeing the future—or a possible future, that is—of an earth that is yet to come, just as soon as the ideas filter through.

On the astral plane we can also visit the Hall of Records, which is like a giant library or video room, where we can explore the history of the world and of our lives to review our "accomplishments" and "failures" and see where we should be going next. We can meet with spiritual teachers and ask them for advice on this too (or on anything else).

You can really explore on the astral in complete freedom and safety, because you cannot be hurt and, wherever you go and whatever you do, you can never get lost or stuck there. For one thing, the astral plane is made up of energy, thoughtforms, and ideas. You are this energy too, and you are the one having the ideas, so, with just a thought, you can bring yourself back to your body any time you wish.

Secondly, there is a cord of energy (some people call it the silver cord) that runs from your solar plexus, like an umbilical cord, to your astral body. This connects you to your physical body and is like an anchor, so there's no way you can float off.

It's also a channel for thought. So just by saying to yourself "I want to go home now," that's what you get! An impulse is sent along the silver cord, and you'll be drawn gently back to earth like you're being reeled in.

So you can explore the astral fearlessly! Millions of people have. They're fine and so will you be. Here's how you get there.

Following Your Dreams

Gine, or the astral plane, is the world of dreams and dreaming. Some Voodoo practitioners say we go there every night as we sleep. To begin exploring astral projection, therefore, first pay attention to your dreams. Remember them as soon as you wake up, then write them down and record them. If anything seems significant about your dream—if some of it leaps out at you or you feel there's a message to it—there probably is, so focus on that.

What does that image mean to you? In 99 percent of cases, there's information in it that will help you with something that's going on in your life. Our spirit guides and ancestors communicate with us in dreams and give us the tools we need to make our lives more perfect.

By working with dreams, you'll be enhancing your creative abilities and imaginative powers as well. Dancing, painting, writing, poetry, or music—any creative activities, in fact—are good for this too. Walking in nature, meditating, and journeying—and, of course, good old-fashioned sex—will also get you out of your body and help you develop these powers, so use them all to expand your mind.

Then try active dreaming. Lie down in your temple and get yourself nicely relaxed. Make sure you're warm and comfortable and you won't be disturbed for an hour or so. Then let yourself drift—not fully off to sleep, but into that sort of drowsy, dreamy, half-in and half-out state of light trance. When you feel this drowsiness, set yourself an intention to visit a place or time or person on the astral plane. Follow the pictures, feelings, or words that pop into your mind when you've done that, and let things unfold naturally like you're watching a film.

After a little while of this, start to direct things a bit more. If you're watching a scene of two people talking, for example, go over and join in, and see if the action or the topic of conversation changes as you influence events. Keep this practice up for a while; once a day, say, for a period of a month or so.

Now comes the fun part! Once you've got the hang of this, find someone you can do it with. Tell them about astral projection and show them how to do it. There a few good games you can play together then, such as:

Home Visits

Visit your friend's house (or have her visit you) during your dreams. Look around when you get there; see what she's wearing, what ornaments or furniture she has out, what book's lying next to her bed, and so on. (If you're too familiar with her house layout in ordinary reality, ask her to move something or make a few other changes. Do the same at your place too.) When your astral travels are over, phone each other or meet up for coffee and talk about your experiences. See if you spotted the changes your friend made or can tell her what she was wearing. You might not get it all 100 percent correct the first few times, but your powers will quickly develop and soon you'll notice improvements.

Hide and Go Seek

Ask your friend to hide on the astral plane, choosing anywhere she likes. It might be a place she's visited and knows from real life, somewhere she's seen on TV, or a fantasy land from a story. Any of these is fine as long as she has a good, clear picture of it. Now track her down by projecting yourself onto the astral and following the trail of her images until you find where she's hiding. When you've found her, bring yourself back to normal consciousness and give her a call. Tell her where she was hiding and listen to her feedback. Then you'll know how accurate you were and give yourself a benchmark for future progress.

Going Out Together

Another option is to travel the astral together. Lie down (side by side or in separate houses) at the same time as your friend and take a tour with the intention that you'll meet up in the otherworld. When you get back, talk to each other and discuss your individual experiences. What do they have in common? What did you see or do? Where did you go, and who was there? Did anyone say anything that you both remember?

Practice, practice, practice! But always have fun and play!

Out-of-Body Sex

And the point of all this practice (well, as far as this chapter goes, anyway) is so you can use astral projection to enjoy a sex life that is *really* out of this world. Once you know how to leave your body, you and your lover can experiment with soul sex, a Voodoo-Tantric practice where, as the name suggests, you meet each other on the astral for sexy times together.

Why would you want to do that? I can think of at least four good reasons.

Firstly, soul sex has a different, more ethereal, deeper quality to it. The physical body can be quite klutzy—has to be positioned right, moved around, and sometimes it takes forever—but things are different on the astral. Here, everything is faster, smoother, easier; all things are possible and can be done with a thought, so sex becomes richer, more intense, and more powerful. Since there's no real time in the otherworld, you can have an orgasm that seems to go on for weeks if that's what you want, or multiple orgasms, one on top of the other, for fifteen years straight. And no sexual position or practice is off-limits if it's something you'd like to try together!

Secondly, because there's no sense of distance or separation in the otherworld, you can have sex together even if you're on different continents. This is something you might have a need for if you're sleepless in Seattle while he's horny in Houston because of that inconvenient business trip!

If you're trying for a baby and monitoring temperatures and times of the month so you know when you're ovulating, it might be important to be able to have long-distance astral sex too. If the moment's absolutely perfect for you to conceive but he's off at a steam enthusiast's rally for the weekend (or doing one of those other really important things men do at times like this), you'll need another way to get hold of his semen pronto. If that sounds a bit bizarre—that you could get pregnant through out-of-body sex—don't dismiss it too quickly. Conceiving a child from the otherworld is an established practice in Buddhism, where they call spirit-babies like this *tulpa*. I don't know what they're called in Voodoo, but I've seen it in Haiti too. And if that doesn't convince you, take a look in the Bible and read how Mary got pregnant by an angel.

Thirdly, while age, health, physical condition, sexual skills, finances, experience, sexual orientation, or any number of things might mean limitations for your sex life in ordinary reality, there are no such problems in the astral world because when you're there, you are what you think and feel.

In your day-to-day life, your sexual preferences or orientation may make it harder for you to find a partner, for example, or ill health may prevent you from having sex or performing as you'd like, but not in Gine, where all things are perfect, everything works, and everyone is young, vital, and available. We all have an inherently sexual nature and urges we must respond to. Astral sex lets us do that, no matter what our ordinary circumstances. Otherworldly sex is very user-friendly!

Finally, Gine, the spirit world, infinity, or the astral—whatever you wish to call it—is made of the energy of love. Love, as the Sisters of the Miracles of Night teach and the priestesses of Aphrodite knew, is the creative force of the universe. When we have sex on the astral plane, we are literally in love, and we make love through our actions. If this idea turns you on, try having sex in paradise!

Here's how you go about it.

Astral Sex for Him

Once he's experienced astral projection and practiced with a friend or two, he'll already know the most important parts of this.

First, make sure he's in the mood. Have him look at a few "dirty" pictures or enjoy a few sexy thoughts. Arousal stirs up our sexual energy and gives new power to the soul. Take him to your temple when you're both ready, and (as best he now can!) ask him to relax into that sleepy, trancelike state. He should then set an intention to visit the astral plane and meet you there.

Tell him to visualize his sexual energies pumping through his energy body and transforming themselves, through serpent flight, into a snakelike extension (a bit like a large penis) that emerges from his genitals. Let his consciousness flow into this new appendage and follow it as it becomes a guided missile taking him into the otherworld (an example of men *really* being led by their penises).

This energy-appendage knows your scent and will lead him to you on the astral plane. It will then naturally and effortlessly enter your vagina and, from there, flow outwards to fill your entire body. As this happens, see how it feels to you.

To him (and to you) it will seem like a blending of sexual energies, so he becomes partly you, which means he'll feel what you're feeling too—a *very* sensual experience! At the same time, he will be intensely aware of his penis and its sensations. He might even feel like that's all there is of him: one giant penis, heightened to vast and exquisite levels!

The intensity of all these lush, new feelings means some men can experience a spontaneous orgasm from this alone, especially if it's their first taste of astral sex. Practice will mean he lasts longer, though, and his sensations will become deeper and even more divine—so tell him to keep it up!

Astral Sex for Her

Women should follow the same initial procedure as men, but visualize your projected self as an extension of your energy body in the shape of snakelike vagina. Take your attention into it and let it lead you to your partner. Your energy-vagina will envelop his penis when you find him and, through this, you will enter his body, where your energy will expand to engulf him.

Again, this feels like a blending of energies, so you experience what it's like to be your lover making love to you while, at the same time, your attention will very definitely be on the heightened sensations in your vagina. Again, it's not unusual for women to orgasm straightaway when this contact is made. As with everything, practice makes it more perfect still!

Astral Sex for You Both

Out-of-body sex is even more intense when you're having physical sex at the same time. Not only is there an energetic connection between you and your lover but a physical one, too, which creates deeply erotic feelings. As you project your etheric vagina into your lover (in the way described above) and merge with his energy body, you become one entity endlessly making love. It's like having sex with yourself and with the entire universe all at once, in a way that is much deeper and more passionate than any sex you've ever had before—with yourself or anyone else!

Sèk limyè—the energy centers of your body—are also triggered when energies combine, and a flood of male and female sexual energies will be exchanged between you, especially at the genitals. This feels like a massive sexual arousal on a scale you'll never have experienced before. Your sensitivity increases by about 1,000 percent so it's like you actually *become* your genitals. Your erogenous zones wake up and start singing all over your body; even your skin feels alive, and touching and being touched will both give you an exquisite thrill!

Because you are sharing the energy body of your lover, your connection becomes even more powerful and you will discover a telepathic link between you. You will feel his experiences and emotions, hear his erotic thoughts, and know exactly what to do to pleasure him because it'll feel like pleasuring yourself.

As your lovemaking reaches its climax, you will have *two* orgasms—not the usual one if you're lucky—physical *and* energetic. If you time this so they occur simultaneously, it can be truly mind-blowing!

Oh yes, there's a lot to be said for astral sex! If you have no other interest in Voodoo, and no desire to learn any other spiritual technique, this is the one you *don't* want to miss!

Sex with the Gods

Another way that astral travel can be used in Voodoo is to have sex with the *lwa* themselves as a blending of their energies with yours. This is a form of *maryaj-lwa*, or "marriage to the spirits." By journeying to Gine, where the *lwa* live, you can offer yourself as a sexual partner and find a spirit-husband or spirit-wife from among the gods.

During astral sex, we merge with our lovers and become them as we share their energies. *Maryaj-lwa* is the same, except that, for a time, we become *gods*. When we blend with Ogoun (the spirit of power), Erzulie (the spirit of love), or Loko or Ayizan (the first priest and priestess of Voodoo), we know what they know, feel what they feel, and embody the qualities they represent.

The procedure is exactly the same as that above: relax in your temple, set your intention to meet a particular *lwa* and to offer yourself in sexual union, then let your energy guide you where you need to go.

Because you are meeting a *lwa*, however—an angel, or an aspect of divine energy—and not just Joe Blow the pizza delivery boy, you will, of course, be respectful at all times, and you'll have done your homework first!

Journey to the *lwa* of your choice a few times, get to know them, and do some research on them (there's more information in my book *Va-Va-Voodoo* and in my colleague's book *Vodou Shaman*) before you throw yourself at them. The gods of Voodoo enjoy sex as much as anyone and know the value of creative union, so they're unlikely to turn you down, but etiquette dictates that if you wouldn't just chuck your panties at Pierce Brosnan (even if he is dishy), you wouldn't do it to Ogoun either!

Also, since you're asking for something from the spirit you blend with—that they give you a part of their power—the first thing you'll want to do is make an offering to them. A plate of their favorite foods with a candle in the appropriate color and prayers that they hear your request are the minimum requirement here before you take off on any out-of-body journey and expect a god to simply show up!

Having said all that, a partnership like this with the spirits is not that unusual in Haiti, and it helps the *lwa* do their work as well. The essence of the *lwa* and of the universe is *love*, but because we don't always get that message, the spirits are happy to find human partners who do and through whom they can spread their loving message.

Remember that it *is* a partnership, though, so there are things you'll need to do, too, as your side of the bargain. One of these is to remain true to the spirit you marry. This doesn't mean you can never have sex with anyone else again, but it *may* mean that one night a week you sleep alone in a separate bed where your spirit-lover can visit you (they come in dreams, so be alert to the meaning

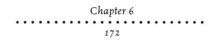
of any you have), that you feed them often, and that they're in your thoughts. It's just like having a regular but not so demanding husband who also gives you something in return!

When you merge with the *lwa*, he or she will tell you how to serve them and how they will serve you in return. I wish you a long and happy marriage!

Grounding Yourself

After any out-of-body experience, it's important to bring yourself fully back to where you belong: planet Earth!

Astral projection is a discipline, something to be done with a purpose and intention in mind, not as a form of escapism and not always just for kicks. You need to have a reason for it and for it to have a beginning and end.

Some of the ways you can get yourself back after astral sex include:

The Ritual Bath

Limes and salt are the key ingredients. Add these to a lukewarm bath and soak in it for fifteen minutes. To this add any other herbs you need to get your energy balanced and flowing again. Grapefruit or black pepper are both good for bringing your attention back to your body (a few drops of either as aromatherapy oils will produce a prickly sensation on your skin so you know you're in the physical rather than the spiritual world); mint is a good oil for "clearing your head" and refreshing you; stone root (*Collinsonia canadensis*—also known as horseweed, richleaf, heal-all, or oxbalm) will add "weight" to your body and give you an anchor to physical reality.

Rocks and Stones

Get yourself three heavy rocks and place one between your feet and another in each hand. Sit with them for ten to fifteen minutes, and they'll "weigh you down" and draw your energy back in to your body. Stamp your feet a few times after this, clap your hands to get your energy flowing again, and drink plenty of water.

Visualization

Focus on your feet. Wiggle your toes and move your feet and ankles. Then do the same with your lower legs, your knees, thighs, hips, genitals, stomach, torso, arms and shoulders, neck, face, and head. Scan yourself thoroughly, and don't feel as if you need to rush anything. Breathe deliberately and slowly throughout the whole process, then take a couple of faster, deeper breaths at the end before you stand up and shake yourself down.

Back in the Physical World:
Food, Sex, and Diet

While we're talking about *energy* bodies, it's worth stating the obvious here: that we get our sexual energy from a variety of sources, and one of them is food. Casanova shared oysters with his women to get them in the mood for love. In the temples of Aphrodite, nuts and seeds (even their names sound sexy) and exotic fruits dripping honey and rich, ripe juices were presented to guests before their other hungers were satisfied. Gran Bwa (the *lwa* of the forests and nature's bounty), Azaka (the spirit of the land), and La Sirène (the goddess of the sea) are all generous with their gifts, and the erotic power of their harvest has been celebrated in Voodoo for centuries.

Many of us in the West don't realize the sexual power of food—until, that is, we stop and reflect for a moment on how many of our erotic encounters began with a dinner for two, and how many special occasions still begin with a quiet restaurant, a corner table, and long, lingering looks over a smouldering candle flame. Food can be sexual magic!

Following the Doctrine of Signatures (see *Va-Va-Voodoo*), foods with sexual power usually resemble genitalia. Gran Bwa stamps his signature on them so we're in no doubt what they're there for! Try licking an oyster out of its shell or sucking a chocolate popsicle and tell me (a) there's nothing else going through your mind, and (b) that if you pay attention, there's not at least a little tingle in your loins as you slurp and suck away.

What we're beginning to find out these days is that Gran Bwa was right to favor sexually powerful foods! Just about every aphrodisiac you can think of is also rich in vitamins and minerals that increase sexual health and potency. The look of the food tells you what it's good for, just as the Doctrine of Signatures predicts. You can, of course, use this in your sexual adventures.

To set the table for love, little "taster" dishes are best, made up of flavors to savor. To enhance the mood, choose foods you can feed each other. Mix and match, and remember it's not just about taste; looks and ambience count too. So select foods that match your intention and communicate your desires to your lover. Some of Gran Bwa's aphrodisiac ingredients for love that you might try are:

Vegetables: Asparagus, artichokes, carrots, celery, cucumbers, mushrooms, olives, radishes, tomatoes, and truffles.

Fruits: Avocados, bananas, dates, figs, mangoes, passion fruit, peaches, pomegranates, and strawberries.

Nuts: Almonds, chestnuts, coconuts, pine, pistachios, and walnuts.

Spices and Herbs: Basil, cardamom, cinnamon, ginger, nutmeg, sage, thyme, and vanilla.

All of these enhance libido, get you in the mood, and give you the energy to follow through.

But, of course, it's not just a case of making a meal out of as many of these things as possible. A little knowledge of nutrition can play an important part in your lovemaking too, as well as the quality of your sex life.

Carbohydrates (found in cereals, pasta, noodles, and sweet potatoes, for example) are your main allies for a lifetime of magical sex, while proteins (especially those in red meats) should only comprise around 20 percent of your daily calorie intake—which is just about the opposite of a typical Western diet! Fried foods, rich sauces, too much sugar, salt, saturated fat, and processed foods leave us feeling sluggish rather than sexual and are linked to heart attacks, frigidity, problems reaching orgasm, and lack of interest in sex. So, a piece of advice: skip the burger on your way to that hot date.

These are the rules if you want to explore the foods of love.

Frolic with Fruit!

Fruits are bubbling with fiber and antioxidants, and give you a burst of energy to deal with even the most demanding lover. Pick up any erotic classic, and you'll find someone, somewhere, feeding someone else a fig, pomegranate, or date—then read on and see what happens next! The people in these stories know what they're doing. Share a passion fruit or a kumquat with your lover, and you'll both receive a burst of juicy energy—and the very act of sharing it together and lapping up all those juices will give you a good idea of how to put that energy to use!

Veg equals Va-Va-Voom!

A lot of vegetables are phallic—asparagus, corn, and carrots among them—and all of them are, not so coincidentally, packed with vitamins and minerals. The "love apple" (or tomato), for example—a perfect little fruity testicle if ever I saw one—is full of lycopene, which is a libido enhancer and works wonders for testes. Never underestimate the Doctrine of Signatures or the sexual power of an artichoke!

Fish for It!

Shellfish fuel the body and pump up the sex drive. Oysters, for example—one of our greatest aphrodisiacs—are packed with zinc, a vital sexual nutriment and essential for testosterone production.

Beef Up Your Meat!

Lean white meats such as chicken and turkey are full of protein and low on fats. Red meats are okay in moderation but shouldn't form a part of every meal as they can clog things up and leave you feeling heavy and bloated. Whenever you can, choose organic meats to avoid hormones, antibiotics, and other nasty additives that do you no good at all.

Don't Forget Your Vitamins!

A natural, healthy diet will give you all the sexual stamina you need. Unfortunately, however, unless you're growing your own organic, genetically unmodified, and chemical-free food, you can't rely on any food to be natural or healthy these days, so it will pay off to take a few vitamin and mineral supplements if you want to be tip-top for sex. The best ones to go for are vitamins A, B, C, and E. All of them aid what scientists call "sexual functioning"—or, in plain terms, they help you get it on. Vitamin E supplies oxygen to the genitals; B improves stamina; selenium aids sexual interest and drive; and zinc gives you added zing. You can take any of these individually according to what you need, or, simpler still, take them all together as multivitamins so they can perk you up in general.

For more information on diet, check appendix 1 at the back of this book.

A Ritual Picnic for the God of the Forest

This is a ritual of thanks to Gran Bwa, who has provided healing herbs and the plants, nuts, and fruits of the forest that give us our natural energy for sex.

Start by selecting foods that are as fresh, organic, and natural as possible. Choose a mixture of different nibbles—a little of this, a little of that—and add one or two more exotic things, like truffles, oysters, and champagne, so you make this a real celebration. A cocktail of erotic fruits, like grapes, mango, passion fruit, and lychees; vegetables whose shapes stimulate your imagination, like asparagus and celery; almonds for sexual energy; and juices, like cranberry and mango, are good to include as well. Foods that melt, drip, and smear, like cream, mayonnaise, and chocolate, are excellent choices too.

Make these up as a picnic, taking your time to appreciate the foods you are including, each of which is a gift to you, through Gran Bwa, from the goddess herself. Have your lover with you as you prepare this feast, but don't let him help; this is your chance to be a priestess and to serve him. You can create a nice sexual tension as you do this by preparing it in the nude. Or perhaps wear just a skimpy apron, and use your striptease skills to tantalize your man—but, again, don't let him touch. The idea is to raise the temperature, but not too far—yet.

When everything is ready, get dressed and take a drive to the country, somewhere quiet where you won't be disturbed. Now, by "get dressed," I don't mean for Arctic conditions. In fact, one very sexy thing you can do is wear stockings, a long coat—and nothing else (don't tell your lover you've done this, though; all he should know is you're going on a picnic).

The *vever* for Gran Bwa is a leaf in a humanlike shape, with erect and fertile plants growing around him, demonstrating the spiritual and sexual powers of the forest and the foods it provides us with:

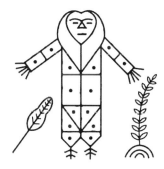

Gran Bwa is there in the trees and leaves, so find yourself a beautiful tree to sit under and spread your picnic blanket on the ground beneath it. Decorate your "table" with flowers, pine cones, leaves, and other plants gathered from the forest, and, if you've brought a green candle with you for Gran Bwa, make this your centerpiece and light it (safely, of course, so you don't start a forest fire; that's *not* what I mean by "raising the temperature"!) .

Raise your food basket to the four directions to receive the blessings of the *lwa*, and thank Gran Bwa for the creative and sexual powers his food gives you, for your lover, for yourself, and for the pleasure of being alive.

You and your partner can now enjoy your food in a playful, loving way, and with an awareness of the sexual charge between you. Sip your fruit juice or champagne from a single glass (very sensual); serve him finger foods, like salty olives or raw vegetables and dip (which gives you the opportunity to "slip" once in a while and smear mayo or cream on his lips, which you can then lick off); feed him a juicy slice of mango, popping it into his mouth with your tongue.

Finally, make yourself the dessert! When the moment is right and all that sensual food has put you in the mood, open your coat to reveal what you're (not) wearing beneath it. Clear away the picnic and use the blanket for other purposes!

Look around you as you make love; let your spirit blend with the forest, and be grateful for all you have and for all you are. Your appreciation of life is the greatest gift you can offer the *lwa* for all they give to you!

Completely in the Dark about Sex

Part of my initiation into Voodoo was to be blindfolded and placed in the *djevo*, the heart of the Voodoo temple, where no light penetrates, and to remain like that for the best part of a week. Pretty dull, you might think, but mystics the world over have used darkness in this way to let go of the world outside and, through that, to find enlightenment. Some remarkable things happen! As the Chinese sage Lao-Tsu wrote, darkness can be "the gateway to all understanding."

Being in the dark for some time brings about a stillness of mind from which intuition, creativity, and new levels of dream consciousness can arise. The imagination is set free and reaches out to the spirits, who bring us their gifts of insight. Those in the *djevo* become *seers*: people who know the world not through their eyes, but with their entire bodies. Our other senses become heightened as well. Hearing becomes more acute; the breeze on the skin feels like satin; if there are others in the *djevo* with us, we can tune in to them so we know their thoughts and feelings.

There's another reason why darkness enhances our sensory and psychic abilities. The brain produces melatonin and pinoline in darkness, biochemicals that create natural dreaming states, as well as DMT, which is one of the active ingredients in many hallucinogenic plants. We feel dreamy, spacey—and sexy!

As an added bonus, it's also said that the nectars of the body take on a hypnotic quality when you use them in magic after being in darkness for some time, because of the dreamy DMT that floods your body. Through the use of darkness-infused nectars it is possible, among other things, to make anyone fall hypnotically in love or in lust with you. They will feel like they have no choice.

You don't even need to be in darkness long for all this to happen. Sometimes a few hours are enough.

As part of *your* initiation into goddess energy, choose a time with your lover, of, say, two or three hours, during which you will both wear blindfolds and stay in your darkened temple. You can build up to longer periods if you wish.

Tune in to each other as you lie in the darkness and explore each other's bodies with your senses: How does your lover's skin feel? What is his scent and his natural odor? What does his breathing tell you about him? How does he taste? Make love in the darkness and open to new sensations and knowledge.

When you take off your blindfolds and look at each other, what do you *see*? Do things look different now that your eyes are truly opened and you have become sexual seers?

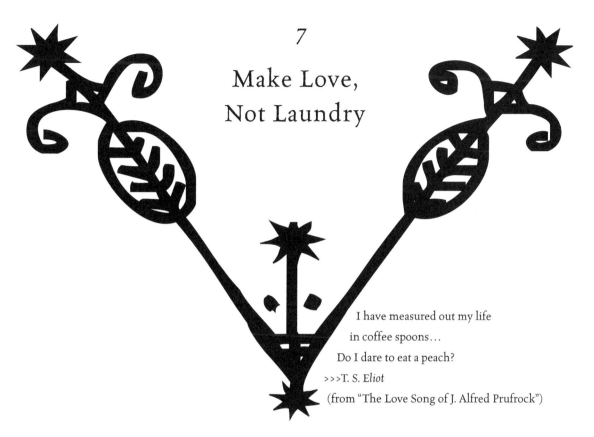

7

Make Love,
Not Laundry

I have measured out my life

in coffee spoons…

Do I dare to eat a peach?

>>>T. S. *Eliot*

(from "The Love Song of J. Alfred Prufrock")

This chapter is a final plea for sanity in a world gone mad—and to encourage you to take up the mantle as a sacred slut and modern goddess!

How many coffee spoons have you gone through in your life, and how many peaches have you eaten?

This mad world we live in is one of endless distractions—trains to catch, jobs to get, promotions to earn, dinner parties to give, deadlines to meet, TV to watch, the laundry to do, coffees to drink, and spoons to line up—but most of it's just filling time.

What would happen to the world if we stopped? Not very much. Life would still go on, because there are always other people to catch trains and line up their spoons instead. But what would happen to us? Well, we might get a life and remember what's important: living!

When we fill our days with distractions, it's easy to forget how fragile life is: how frail and in need of love we are, and how quickly all this will be over.

We protect ourselves from those truths with modern rituals of competition, conflict, and warfare—the very opposite of what we are here for and what the spirits want us to do, which is to love, be loved, and to heal!

To make ourselves feel safe, we demand that others are exactly like us and listen to the words of self-appointed moral leaders who tell us that sex is dirty, that creativity is wrong, that love is misguided, and that anyone who is unique and stands in their power is someone we should be afraid of.

If we go along with all this and deny ourselves pleasure, scared of what the consequences might be, what's the point in being alive?

When we don't allow ourselves the delight and the right to have sex, for example—which is, after all, the most natural thing in the world—we're really sending a bigger message. We're saying to ourselves and others "I'm wrong for having sexual feelings—and so are you!" But if that's the case, then God/Goddess must be wrong for giving us these feelings in the first place. And if God/Goddess is wrong (or doesn't really exist), what does it matter what we do? We might as well create hate and chaos in the world.

We have to get beyond this psychology and, as the Sisters of the Miracles of Night teach their disciples, realize that sex can unite us and overcome opposition. The sanctity of human contact is our way back to connection, to peace on earth, and to finding the goddess again. This is why the sisters are the protectors of the "miracles of night" and why they preserve the mysteries of the Horae in secret: so that sex can never be appropriated by the powers-that-be and used against the people.

The Sisters of the Miracles of Night know that the *lwa want* us to be happy. They *want* us to be sacred channels for the creative divine and to serve the goddess with our bodies, because through this, love and healing are spread throughout the world.

So remember what is important. Don't lose yourself in distractions or let the moralists tell you what's right and wrong or that sex is bad. You already know the *real* truth in your soul, because your soul *is* goddess energy. That's the stuff you are made from!

Use your time here to make love, not laundry or lines of coffee spoons—and definitely not war! The greatest thing you can do for this world is to become a goddess and to use your creative brilliance and your body to spread love and happiness with wild, rambunctious, ravenously passionate, juicy, luscious, soul-saving sex!

The Presentation to the Sun

The sun is an incredibly important symbol in Voodoo and represents All-That-Is. Voodoo symbols tend to have Catholic "masks" to keep them secret, so the sun is known as Saint Thomas: the holy man who was the only witness to the ascension of the Virgin Mary into heaven.

When new priests and priestesses leave the *djevo*, the place where they have been secluded in darkness (see chapter 6), they are ritually presented to the sun before they do anything else. They must gaze upwards, like Thomas did, bow to the sun, and give thanks for life.

This simple little ceremony is one of the most crucial (and secret) in Voodoo because it contains cosmic information about the true nature of life. What does it all mean?

In Voodoo, the most important *lwa* is Legba, the sky father and gatekeeper between the worlds of heaven and earth. Legba *is* life, rebirth, and regeneration. One of his symbols is the phallus. Another is the sun. And one of his "masks" is Saint Thomas.

Erzulie is the earth mother, the goddess of love and the muse of beauty. Her "mask" is the Virgin Mary, who ascended into heaven.

When the Voodoo priestess looks at the sky, she sees the blending of male and female energies, sun and moon, Legba and Erzulie, together representing the goddess.

It is this blending of male and female that is the true secret to life. And how do male and female energies blend best? Through sex: the union of Legba and the "ascended" Virgin, the woman who goes beyond her limitations or those imposed upon her.

The sun is Legba and also the pregnant, full belly from which all life comes through growth and fecundity on earth and the harvest of its fruits. The moon is Erzulie and also the moon time of every woman, whose menstrual nectar gives birth to new ideas and energies through the gateway she represents.

When she leaves the *djevo*, the Voodoo priestess is reborn from darkness into light and to the knowledge that sex is precious, natural, and holy. Without it our world could not exist, but through it all miracles are possible.

To symbolize this, the priestess receives mass when she emerges from the *djevo*, but she does not eat "the body of Christ." She is given bread, which comes from Legba, whose sun makes the harvest possible. The bread has been soaked in wine and the red juice of fruits, to symbolize the life-blood of Erzulie and the power of woman and the moon. This sacrament is the union of male and female.

This is a ritual you should also now do.

The Union of the Sun and the Moon

Prepare a sacrament by adding two drops of cinnamon oil to one drop each of rosemary, jasmine, and sandalwood oils in a cup of almond base oil, and use this to anoint a white bowl by lightly smearing the oil around it.

This mixture is a blend of Moon Oil (traditionally used to induce psychic dreams, to increase fertility and sexual passion, and for other lunar influences) and Sun Oil (for vitality, strength, arousal, and solar influences). You'll have plenty left over, which you can store in a dark, cool place and use as a massage oil for temple workings.

Into this bowl place four small pieces of freshly baked bread, and drizzle them with a mixture of red wine, rum, blackcurrant juice, and liquid honey. Let it stand for a few hours until the bread absorbs the mixture and goes red, soggy, and delicious!

When the sun is at its highest, take your sacrament outside and stand in the sun's rays with your lover. Look at the world, the sky, and feel the heat of the sun on your face and the ground beneath your feet.

Turn to your lover and feed him a piece of the bread. Say:

> *For the sun, for the sky, for the goddess*
> *For the soul, for the body, for the power of sex*
> *For the moon, for the earth, for all its richness*
> *This is my body, my blood, my life*
> *This is the way and the end of strife*
> *This is the staff and the holy knife*

The final line refers to Legba, who is often depicted as a man carrying a staff or a cane, and to Erzulie, whose *vever* can be drawn as a sacred heart pierced by a knife.

Your lover repeats these words as he then feeds you.

The Journey to the Sun and the Moon

Following this ceremony, the priestess is given a new, secret name to represent the change she has gone through as a result of her initiation into goddess energy and the knowledge she now has. This is the *nom vanyon*—the "valiant" or "sacred name."

To give her this name, her initiator will journey to the heart of the sun and the moon, the blending of cosmic energies, and *become* the essence of Erzulie and Legba, the combined goddess, so she can look back to earth and see the new priestess standing there. From this, she will know the name to give.

Sacred names represent something about the person named and could translate, for example, as "Stands Defiant" or "Knows the Mysteries of Gine," or something similar. They are usually kept very secret.

This is a ceremony you should now perform. Journey (see chapter 1) to Legba and Erzulie (depicted as the sun and the moon combined, or one behind the other), and let their energies fill you. Then look back to Earth and see yourself. What qualities do you have—or *wish* to have? Who are you, and what is your sacred purpose? As you ask these questions, a form of words will come to you from which your sacred name can be made.

When you have it, bring yourself back to consciousness and whisper your name to the breeze. You can, if you wish, share this name with your lover, or you may choose to keep it secret, just between you and the goddess.

Either way, you should both now light a white candle (one each) in the bowl and offer the two remaining pieces of bread in thanks to Legba and Erzulie, the combined goddess.

Know that you are love, know that you are loved, know that you are special, and know the sacred nature of sex. Then embrace your lover—and your destiny—and get out there and be a sacred goddess slut!

appendix 1

The Voodoo "Detox Diet"

Special detox food is given to initiates in the *djevo* to purify the body and spirit for magical work. Some of these foods are impossible to get in the West and, in any case, the specific "food of Gine" fed to priests and priestesses is highly secret and known to initiates only. But I do advise practitioners and clients to detox if they are working with the body's energies, for example, in sexual healing or preparations involving the nectars.

The detox program below is based on Voodoo and shamanic dieting practices for purification. It changes the energies of the body, mind, spirit, and emotions, leading to greater well-being, balance, and insight, and the ability to let go of unhappy events, issues, and attachments that are causing illness or distress. The shamans say that, through this diet, we remember who we are: children of nature and the goddess.

Procedure

- Follow the diet for a minimum of three days and an absolute maximum of fourteen, but cut it back or stop it completely if you feel any ill effects

- Take a hot bath every day, adding fresh ginger and one drop of black pepper aromatherapy oil (except on the last day)

- On the last day of your diet, break the regime in the evening by drinking the juice of one lemon with a little salt; also take a warm bath with lemon, salt, and rose petals

Foods You Can Eat

Fruits: Most fruits, as well as fruit juices, are okay, but some only in moderation—see below.

Vegetables: Raw or cooked. Good detox vegetables include red and green ones like broccoli, cauliflower, sprouts, onions, garlic, artichokes, and beets. Artichokes increase the flow of bile and help to digest fats. Beets help regenerate liver cells and are good for fat metabolism. Broccoli (and other brassicas like cabbage, cauliflower, sprouts, and kale) support the liver's detoxification enzymes. Onions and garlic are good for sulfation, the main detox pathway for environmental chemicals, drugs, and food additives. They also help with the elimination of heavy metals from the body.

Beans: Split yellow and green peas and lentils are easiest to digest and require the least soaking time. Others include kidney beans, pinto beans, mung beans, chickpeas, and adzuki beans.

Meat: Fish, turkey, chicken.

Rice: Brown or basmati, rice cakes, rice crackers, and rice pasta.

Grains: Quinoa, millet, and buckwheat can be used instead of rice.

Nuts: Unsalted nuts and seeds can generally be eaten. Flaxseed, pumpkin seeds, sesame seeds, sunflower seeds, almonds, cashews, and walnuts are all okay in moderation, but avoid peanuts, which are ritually prohibited during spiritual work like this in Voodoo.

Drinks: Water, herbal drinks and teas, green tea, fruit juice, vegetable juices, and smoothies. No milk.

Any of these foods, raw or simply prepared (e.g., steamed, boiled, or grilled), can be combined, and in any quantities you wish, although it is best not to eat too much and to skip the evening meal and just eat raw snack foods after about 6 PM. The key is simple food, simply prepared. Go for the freshest organically grown and additive-free foods you can.

Foods to Avoid

Salt: Salt, like limes and lemons, is said to "cut through magic," and the spirits are repelled by it. However, this must be tempered by common sense. Human beings do require an intake of salt, and prolonged periods without it can lead to illness. Most foods naturally contain enough salt, but if you need a little more, add it in moderation. To give you an idea of how little you may need, the addition of a single olive each day is probably enough.

Oils and fats.

Spices.

Lemon and lime.

Pork and pork fats or additives derived from pork (check labels).

Alcohol.

Soy beans and soy products: Such as soy sauce, tofu, miso, and teriyaki.

Excess meat and especially red meats.

Sauces: These generally contain spices, salts, and citrus ingredients, all of which are prohibited, so check the contents or avoid.

Refined sugar and mixtures containing refined sugar: Including sucrose, dextrose, corn syrup, and brown sugar. Also avoid artificial sweeteners.

Wheat and products containing wheat.

Gluten: Including that in grains such as barley and rye.

Yeast.

Chocolate.

Processed foods in general.

Foods You Can Eat in Moderation (e.g., Once a Week)

Fruits: Avocado, eggplant, figs, grapes, oranges, pineapple, plums, prunes, raisins.

Dairy: Butter, yogurt, cheese (cottage cheese only), skim milk. But, in general, avoid dairy products.

Bread: Dry—no butter or spreads.

Dietary Dos and Don'ts

Do drink a minimum of eight glasses of water a day, warm or at room temperature, to clear waste from the blood.

Do dilute fruit juice with 50 percent water.

Do chew food well, especially grains.

Do avoid recreational drugs.

Do begin a practice of daily meditation during the diet, and take walks in nature so you slow down to the pace of the natural world.

Don't drink anything at or around mealtimes.

Don't take part in loud and frenetic social gatherings.

Don't watch too much TV, listen to loud music, or get involved in other distractions. The idea is to free yourself as much as possible from attachments so you create a space for your spirit to flow.

Helpful Herbs and Vitamins

Dandelion root increases the flow of bile.

Milk thistle has positive effects on the liver. It is an antioxidant, assists in liver cell regeneration, and neutralizes adverse effects from alcohol or fat consumption.

Multivitamins containing selenium, molybdenum, and zinc are good for energy rebalancing.

Vitamin C is an antioxidant that also helps reduce some side effects of detox, such as headache or nausea.

Protein is required by the liver for detox and is found in fish, beans, nuts, seeds, quinoa, etc.

And, of course, *always* check with your doctor before you begin a diet like this!

appendix 2

Aphrodisiacs, Perfumes, Bath Oils, and Essences to Make Him Go "Ooh"

Aphrodisiacs are sexual stimulants named after Aphrodite (Erzulie), the goddess of sex, love, and beauty—and there are hundreds of them! The world is teeming with sex.

Foods

Voodoo's Doctrine of Signatures tells us that aphrodisiacs are obvious from their looks, and this is how they have usually developed their legendary status. Oysters look, smell, feel, and sometimes taste like little vaginas, for example; ginseng (which means "man root") looks like a small man, complete with bumps in all the right places, and even tastes a little musky.

Other aphrodisiacs get their reputations from the effect they have on us (chilies and other spicy foods get our pulses racing and make us "hot," for example) or because of their rarity, value, and mystery. Chocolate was once the ultimate turn-on because of its exotic origins and its unusual taste and texture, but its reputation began to wear off when it became more easily available. Even so, scientists tell us that chocolate releases exactly the same chemicals in our brains that we produce during sex—proof that our ancestors knew what they were doing when they were licking chocolate body paint off each other while huddled round a cave fire!

Aphrodite was born from the sea, and most seafoods therefore have a reputation as aphrodisiacs. Oysters are the classic amorous dish to serve, but all fish contain the "brain food" omega-3 to keep us energized, awake, and up for it, and shellfish are rich in zinc, which increases sex drive and passion.

Here are a few aphrodisiac recipes you can try.

Seafood Special

Take six raw oysters and add three drops of Tabasco (more if you like it hot) and a little chili, a diced spring onion, and a chopped stick of celery (all of them aphrodisiacs in their own right).

Put all the ingredients in a blender and add a dash of brandy, a little horse-radish, and a few spoons of sour cream, then blend to make a sauce. Throw in a few prawns, mussels, and a little crab meat, and warm in a saucepan.

Use this to dress fresh salmon, asparagus, and roasted sweet potatoes. Serve to your lover with a crisp white wine, and watch him turn to putty in your hands!

Vegetable Surprise

The surprise is the effect it has! Roughly chop mushrooms, tomatoes, and onions, and fry till soft in a little olive oil. Transfer to a baking dish and add sweet corn, spinach, and sautéed potatoes.

Spice with a little basil, tamarind, a bay leaf, a pinch of five-spice, and a little French mustard. Add a sauce made with white wine and cream, and coat with grated Cheddar cheese. Then cook in a moderate oven until the cheese forms a crust. Serve hot.

Fruit Medley

The simpler the better with fruit, because the goodness (and the goddess) is already in it. Just add fresh dates, figs, mangoes, peaches, and sliced strawberries to a bowl and sprinkle with almonds, coconut flakes, or pomegranate seeds.

A spoon or two of chocolate mousse on top never hurt either, and grated dark chocolate makes a finishing touch.

Oils and Essences

Aphrodisiacs aren't just foods, though. In Voodoo there's an art to blending oils, bath essences, and perfumes that also have aphrodisiac qualities. Most of the ingredients are easy enough to get hold of, and the potions are quick and easy to make. Here are a few for your sexual armory. (For more, see *Va-Va-Voodoo*.)

Sexy Perfume

Add a handful of fragrant rose petals, half a tablespoon of cloves, two crushed bay leaves, a small piece of fresh ginger, a pinch of yohimbe, one drop of bergamot oil, and one drop of frankincense to a cup of white wine vinegar. Bring this to a boil in a saucepan, and simmer for ten minutes.

Take it off the heat and leave it to cool, then strain it into a dark bottle with a good stopper to it. Blow your intention for love and sex into it, and let it stand for at least two weeks before you use it.

Sexy Bath Essence

Take petals of musk roses, carnations, jasmine, and geranium, and add a few sprigs of mint and lemon verbena, then roughly chop them all together. Put these in a jar and add a sliver of soap and a dash of Florida water or white rum, then fill up to the top with spring water. Blow in your intention.

Put the lid on the jar and leave it in a warm room for nine days, giving it a shake every now and then and each time before you use it. Add some to your bath water and take a relaxing candlelit soak to activate its magic.

Sexy Oils

These come from Hoodoo, a form of Voodoo popular in the southern United States. The first is called Aphrodite Oil, and as the name suggests, it's a natural aphrodisiac; the second is for sexual energy. You can use them both in oil burners in your temple, wear them like a perfume on the pulse points at your wrists and throat, or add them to bath water for a stimulating soak.

Aphrodite Oil: Add five drops of cypress and two drops of cinnamon aromatherapy oils to a cupful of olive base oil. To this add a small piece of orris root (this is the root of some iris species grown in southern Europe), and pour it into a dark bottle and seal it. Leave it for nine days to mature, then use it freely.

Serpent Flight Oil: Add two drops of ginger, two of patchouli, and one each of cardamom and sandalwood to a half cup of olive base oil. Pour the mixture into a dark bottle, seal it, and leave it for nine days before use.

appendix 3

Your Sexual Compatibility Chart

Voodoo has always been a tradition that has borrowed from others. It could hardly be otherwise since it began in Africa, moved to Haiti with the slaves, and got mixed up with a whole lot of European and American shamanic practices, Jewish mysticism, and pagan, Wiccan, and other beliefs en route. Whatever works *works*, after all!

In recent years, as more Westerners visit Haiti and initiate into Voodoo, British and American astrological practices have become popular there as well, and there are now many Voodoo practitioners who are expert star-gazers. You'll remember from the opening chapter that the Horae were the watchers of the stars and keepers of the hours (in fact, the word *horoscope* comes from their temple practices), so it's not surprising that the sisterhood's members are also practiced astrologers.

I'm not going to go into much detail here, however, because I'm *not* an astrologer! And, anyway, there are plenty of other books on the subject. What I do want to give you, though, is this simple chart you can use to predict your sexual compatibility with any new partner who may be coming over your horizon.

Simply check your sign against his and it'll tell you your ideal lover (sexual sparks will fly!), star signs that mix okay with yours, and the ones you'd be better off avoiding because the sex that comes out of it will never set the world on fire.

Your Sign	His Ideal Sign	Okay Signs	Not So Good
Aries	Leo, Libra, Sagittarius	Aquarius, Gemini	Cancer, Capricorn
Taurus	Capricorn, Scorpio, Virgo	Cancer, Pisces	Aquarius, Leo
Gemini	Aquarius. Libra, Sagittarius	Aries, Leo	Pisces, Virgo
Cancer	Capricorn, Pisces, Scorpio	Taurus, Virgo	Aries, Libra
Leo	Aquarius, Aries, Sagittarius	Gemini, Libra	Scorpio, Taurus
Virgo	Capricorn, Taurus	Cancer, Scorpio	Gemini, Pisces, Sag
Libra	Aquarius, Aries, Gemini	Leo, Sagittarius	Cancer, Capricorn
Scorpio	Cancer, Pisces, Taurus	Capricorn, Sag, Virgo	Aquarius, Leo
Sagittarius	Aries, Leo	Aquarius, Libra	Pisces, Virgo
Capricorn	Cancer, Taurus, Virgo	Pisces, Scorpio	Aries, Libra
Aquarius	Gemini, Leo, Libra	Aries, Sagittarius	Scorpio, Taurus
Pisces	Cancer, Scorpio	Capricorn, Taurus	Gemini, Sag, Virgo

But remember, it's just a guide. Don't chuck him out of bed just yet—not until you've seen for yourself if he's beyond your help!

appendix 4

Your Sexual Compatibility Numbers

Another art that has also grown popular in Voodoo is numerology. The simplest way of using this to check your sexual compatibility is to add up the letters in your name and your lover's name and then compare them.

In numerology, all letters of the alphabet are given a value, so A = 1, B = 2, C = 3, all the way through to X (24), Y (25), and Z (26). Voilà!

A	B	C	D	E	F	G	H	I	J	K	L	M
1	2	3	4	5	6	7	8	9	10	11	12	13
N	O	P	Q	R	S	T	U	V	W	X	Y	Z
14	15	16	17	18	19	20	21	22	23	24	25	26

Use this to record the numbers in your name—so, for example:

K	A	T	H	L	E	E	N	C	H	A	R	L	O	T	T	E
11	1	20	8	12	5	5	14	3	8	1	18	12	15	20	20	5

Zeroes don't count and all double numerals should be added together, like this:

K	A	T	H	L	E	E	N	C	H	A	R	L	O	T	T	E
2	1	2	8	3	5	5	5	3	8	1	9	3	6	2	2	5

Now if you add the numbers up, you get 2+1+2+8+3+5+5+5+3+8+1+9+3+6+2 +2+5=70 (I think! Sums were never my strong point!)

Then reduce them further, so you're left with a final figure. In my case, I come out as a 70, but by reducing this as far as I can, I get 7+0 = 7. So my number's 7.

Figure out what yours is, then do the same for your lover. You can then compare and contrast. In terms of sexual compatibility, here's what the figures *could* mean and the numbers who are most likely—and least likely—to give you that earth-shattering orgasm:

YOUR NUMBER	RED-HOT SEX!	NOT BAD IN BED!	SO-SO SEX!	FORGET ABOUT IT!
1	1,5,7	3,9	8	2,4,6
2	2,4,8	3,6	9	1,5,7
3	3,6,9	1,2,5		4,7,8
4	2,4,8	6,7		1,3,5,9
5	1,5,7	3,9	8	2,4,6
6	3,6,9	2,4,8		1,5,7
7	1,5,7	4	9	2,3,6,8
8	2,4,8	6	1,5	3,7,9
9	3,6,9	1,5	2,7	4,8

Take a chart like this for what it is and no more, of course. It's an *indicator* of what's going on and where you could do more to get things cooking—but that's all it is. You know your relationships better than anyone else, and no matter what the numbers say, if the sex works for you, that's *all* you need to know!

Glossary

A short explanation of Voodoo, Haitian, relationship, and sexual psychology terms used in this book. Pronunciation is given where this may be needed.

Ancestors: Known in Voodoo as *zanset yo*—loved ones who have passed over into spirit.

Aphrodisiac: A potion, food, or herb with special powers to raise libido and sexual desire.

Aphrodite: The Greek goddess of love (Voodoo equivalent: Erzulie).

Ashe: (ash-AY) Spiritual power.

Astral body: The energy body (or soul/light body); in Voodoo, the *nanm*.

Astral projection: "Soul flight" or out-of-body travel.

Astral sex: "Soul sex"; the practice of out-of-body sexual relations.

Ayida-Wedo: (i-YAY-DA-WAY-do) The female cosmic serpent who, with her husband, Damballah, gave birth to all life.

Ayizan Velekete: (i-yee-ZAN val-EK-t) The first Voodoo priestess and the mother of initiates; now a *lwa*.

Azaka: (az-AK-ar) The *lwa* of the land.

Banda: The sexy dance practiced by Baron.

Baron: (bar-RON) The *lwa* who is guardian of the cemetery.

Barrier signal: Unconscious body language, like crossed legs or folded arms, that presents a protective front to another.

Binding: A magical spell or Voodoo "trick" to hold another person to you.

Bondye: (bon-DEE) In Voodoo, god—and ultimately goddess— energy. From the French *bon dieu* ("good god").

Brigid: (brij-IT) The *lwa* who is wife to Baron.

Chacapa: (shak-KAP-ah) A special bundle of leaves used in shamanic and Voodoo healing.

Chakras: In Voodoo, *sèk limyè*—energy centers in the body.

Chantes: (shan-TES) Sacred songs used to call the *lwa*.

Curses: Words used to send negative energy toward someone.

Damballah: (DAM-ba-LAH) The male cosmic serpent who, with his wife, Ayida-Wedo, gave birth to all life.

Danse-lwa: (dance-lo-AH) The possession-trance of Voodoo.

Detox: The process of purifying the body and removing toxins, used in shamanic and Voodoo diets; for example, when working with the body's nectars.

Djab: (jab) A Voodoo spirit.

Djevo: (jay-VO) The inner sanctum of the Voodoo temple.

Doctrine of Signatures: The belief that plants, herbs, and foods reveal what they are used for by their appearance; for example, that aphrodisiac foods often resemble genitalia.

Endocrine alchemy: Special Voodoo practices, such as dieting and detox, which produce particular effects in the body.

Energy body: The astral body or soul (*nanm*).

Erogenous zones: Areas of the body that, when stimulated, lead to arousal.

Erzulie: (er-ZOO-LI) The *lwa* of love and luxury.

Expedition: The sending of a spirit, energy, or intention to another person.

Florida water: A special perfume used in Voodoo for cleansing and spellcraft.

Gine: (ginn-AY) The spirit world, or Voodoo heaven.

Gran Bwa: The *lwa* of the forests and nature's bounty.

"Grower": One of two types of penis; nothing to write home about until it is erect.

Hexing: The practice of sending curses or making harmful spells.

Hoodoo: A form of Voodoo popular in the Southern United States.

Horae: The sacred sluts and priestesses in the temples of Aphrodite.

Houngan: (oon-GAN) Voodoo priest.

Infinity symbol: The figure eight, a symbol of power also known as the lemniscate.

Intimate zone: In the psychology of body language, the area closest to us, into which we are usually only comfortable enough to allow our lovers and close friends.

Jing: A concept in Chinese medicine that describes the vital essences, spirit, or energies stored in the body.

Klè dlo: (clay-DA-lo) The "clear waters" (nectars) of the body, such as tears and sweat, that contain emotional energy.

Konfyans: (kon-FI-yonz) The practice of spiritual "confession" or the confessor this is made to.

Kundalini: The coiled serpent energy at the base of the spine.

La Sirène: The *lwa* of the sea.

Legba: The *lwa* who is the gatekeeper between heaven (Gine) and earth.

Lemniscate: The infinity symbol or figure eight, used for summoning power.

Les invisibles: The spirits.

Loko Atissou: The first Voodoo priest and the father of initiates; now a *lwa*.

Lwa: (lo-AH) The angels of Voodoo.

Maji: Magic.

Mambo: Voodoo priestess.

Manman: Mother.

Manman Jenèz: The Genesis Mother; leader of the Sisterhood of the Miracles of Night.

Maryaj-lwa: (marr-IJ-lo-AH) "Marriage to the spirits"; a special Voodoo ceremony where a man or woman takes a spiritual partner from among the *lwa*.

Mitan: Heart.

Nanm: The soul.

Nectar: One of the fluids of the body charged with sexual energy.

Nom vanyon: The "valiant" or "sacred name" received by priests and priestesses after their initiations.

Ogoun: The *lwa* of power.

Peristyle: The Voodoo church.

Personal zone: An area around the body, approximately four feet to eighteen inches from the self, where we are only comfortable to allow people we know well.

Porteau mitan: The post at the center of the Voodoo church, known as the "gateway of the heart."

Possession: A trance state in Voodoo where a *lwa* temporarily takes over the body of one of the faithful.

Postural echo: Sharing body language in common with someone else to show an affinity or connection to them.

Pusanga: "Love medicine" used as a perfume, which has special powers of attraction.

Pwen: A ritual Voodoo power object.

Pythoness: The oracle or seer who uses sexual energy (serpent flight) to make divinations, see the future, and pass on messages from spirit.

Sant: A magical Voodoo perfume.

Sèk limyè: *See* Chakras.

Sè Mirak Lanuit: The Sisterhood of the Miracles of Night; a secret society in Haiti which specializes in Tantric-Voodoo sex magic.

Serpent flight: A Tantric-Voodoo practice for liberating sexual energies to generate personal power.

Shamanic journey: A controlled practice for out-of-body experiences, allowing the soul to visit the spirit world.

"Shower": One of two types of penis—relatively big even when flaccid.

Silver cord: A cord of energy that runs from the solar plexus, like an umbilical cord, to the spiritual body during astral travel.

Social zone: An area around the body, approximately four feet from the self, into which we will allow others during social situations.

Soplada: (sew-PLA-dar) The ritual of blowing intention into a magical potion.

Soul sex: Engaging in sexual relations with someone during astral travel or soul flight.

Thunderstones: Magical stones containing power that were formed during the creation of the universe when Damballah and Ayida-Wedo, the snake gods, had sex and gave birth to all life.

Tulpa: Children created by magical means.

Unbinding: A magical procedure to release two people linked together through the casting of a spell.

Vever: (vee-VAR) Mystical signs used to call the *lwa*.

Vòl nanm: Astral projection or "soul flight."

Voodoo: Also spelled Vodou; the spiritual tradition of Haiti.

Zam: "Weapon"; a colloquial term for the penis in Haitian Kreyol.

Zanset yo: The ancestors in Voodoo; loved ones who have passed over to spirit and are among the most important of our spiritual guides.

Notes, References,
and Further Reading

Chapter 1, The Rise, Fall, and Res-Erection of the Spiritual Slut

The factbites in this chapter and others in this book are from research conducted by Amora, the London Academy of Sex and Relationships, and featured in their fascinating exhibits and displays at the Trocadero in London. Check out their website at www.amoralondon.com and visit them soon!

Leora Tanenbaum's book *Slut! Growing Up Female with a Bad Reputation* (2000) is published by Harper Paperbacks. See http://leoratanenbaum.com/work1.htm for more information.

The poem "Little Gidding," from which the T. S. Eliot quotation comes, can be found in *Four Quartets* (1968), published by Harvest Books.

My book, *Va-Va-Voodoo: Find Love, Make Love, & Keep Love* (2007) has lots more magical spells for love and practical advice on how to find it, and is published by Llewellyn.

For more information on the *lwa* and on Voodoo in general (though he spells it Vodou), I recommend Ross Heaven's book *Vodou Shaman: The Haitian Way of Healing and Power* (2003), published by Destiny Books.

Chapter 2, Building Your Temple of Love

The facts, figures, and research mentioned in this chapter can also be found at Amora, the London Academy of Sex and Relationships: www.amoralondon.com.

Chapter 3, How to Kiss like a Pro (And Other Things Your Body Can Do)

If you'd like to experiment with other sexual positions, the classic reference source is *The Kama Sutra*. There are many versions available in bookstores, but I like *The Photographic "Kama Sutra"* by Linda Sonntag, which actually shows you what's going on! This is published by Hamlyn (2001).

Chapter 4, Getting Your Freak On: Fantasy Favorites and Filthy Language

The information in the first few pages of this chapter is taken from two studies. The first is the *National Health and Social Life Survey* (NHSLS), which was conducted in the early 1990s and interviewed 3,432 women and men aged 18 to 59. The second was a telephone interview by *The Kinsey Institute* of 987 women aged 20 to 65, conducted between 1999 and 2000.

You can find the 2006 MSNBC Interactive sex survey at http://www.msnbc.msn.com/id/12410076 (current as of March 2007).

The *Elle*/MSNBC survey mentioned in this chapter (under the *Talking Dirty* section) is available online at *Elle*/MSNBC.com Sex and Love Survey (current as of March 2007).

The Heyeokah Guru is the author of *Adam and Evil: The God Who Hates Sex, Women, and Human Bodies* (2007), published by Dandelion Books.

Chapter 5, When I Get That Feeling, I Need Sexual Healing

In the section *Goddess Energy in the Body*, I mentioned the books by my colleague, Ross Heaven, which talk about the energy body. Three good ones to look into if you'd like to know more about this are *The Spiritual Practices of the Ninja* (Inner Traditions, 2006), *Plant Spirit Shamanism* (Inner Traditions, 2006), and *The Way of the Lover* (Llewellyn, 2007).

There is more information on thunderstones and some images at the Four Gates Foundation website: www.thefourgates.com. Look under "Healing and Products."

If you'd like to know a little more about the oracles and seership, there's some more information in *Darkness Visible: Awakening Spiritual Light Through Darkness Meditation* by Ross Heaven (Inner Traditions, 2006).

I mentioned the dancer Gabrielle Roth in the *Dirty Dancing* section. Gabrielle has several books and CDs out. A good place to start is her book *Sweat Your Prayers*. This is published by Tarcher (1998).

Laennec Hurbon, the Haitian professor who writes about Voodoo, whom I also mentioned in this section, has a book called *Discoveries: Voodoo: Search for the Spirit* (Harry N. Abrams, 1995).

Chapter 6, *Sex That's Out of This World!*

The study I mentioned that links sex and creativity was covered in a Reuters news story by Patricia Reaney, posted on Tuesday, November 29, 2006, called Creativity Linked to Sexual Success. If you'd like to know more, see http://www.yayhooray.com/thread/66511/Creativity-linked-to-sexual-success.

Index

Free Catalog

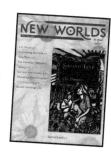

Get the latest information on
our body, mind, and spirit products!
To receive a **free** copy of Llewellyn's consumer
catalog, *New Worlds of Mind & Spirit,* simply call
1-877-NEW-WRLD or visit our website at
www.llewellyn.com and click on *New Worlds.*

LLEWELLYN ORDERING INFORMATION

Order Online:
Visit our website at www.llewellyn.com, select your books, and order them on our
secure server.

Order by Phone:
- Call toll-free within the U.S. at 1-877-NEW-WRLD
  (1-877-639-9753). Call toll-free within Canada at
  1-866-NEW-WRLD (1-866-639-9753)
- We accept VISA, MasterCard, and American Express

Order by Mail:
Send the full price of your order (MN residents add 6.5% sales tax) in
U.S. funds, plus postage & handling to:

> **Llewellyn Worldwide**
> **2143 Wooddale Drive, Dept. 978-0-7387-1200-0**
> **Woodbury, MN 55125-2989**

Postage & Handling:

Standard (U.S., Mexico, & Canada). If your order is:
  $24.99 and under, add $3.00
  $25.00 and over, FREE STANDARD SHIPPING

AK, HI, PR: $15.00 for one book plus $1.00 for
each additional book.

International Orders (airmail only):
  $16.00 for one book plus $3.00 for each additional book

Orders are processed within 2 business days.
Please allow for normal shipping time. Postage and handling rates subject to change.

Va-Va-Voodoo!
Find Love, Make Love & Keep Love
Kathleen Charlotte

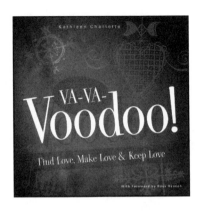

How many professional therapists can put together a powerful mojo bag or an intoxicating love perfume to attract a mate? As a relationship counselor and a Voodoo initiate, Kathleen Charlotte offers the best of both worlds in her refreshing, witty, and magical guide to this crazy little thing called love.

Va-Va-Voodoo introduces five key Voodoo *lwa* or "angels," including Baron, the spirit who loves spicy rum and cigars, and La Sirène, an ocean goddess of seduction and sensuality. Readers learn how to "feed the spirits" and request their help in attracting a lover, finding "the one," keeping a relationship steamy, or recovering from heartbreak. A perfect blend of practical magic and inspiring, down-to-earth advice, this one-of-a-kind book includes magic rituals, charms, aphrodisiacs, and spells, as well as helpful relationship tips regarding communication, self-esteem, intimacy, sex, break-ups, and forgiveness.

0-7387-0994-8, 216 pp., 7 x 7, 2-color interior $14.95

Witch in the Bedroom

Proven Sensual Magic

Stacey Demarco

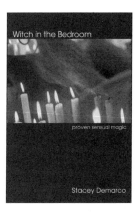

Stacey Demarco brings the "Witch's Way" into the bedroom in this delightful guide to love, sex, and fertility. Blending personal empowerment techniques, core values of Wicca, sex magic, and proven spells, she tackles affairs of the heart with witchy flair.

Demarco begins by tracing the origins of Witchcraft and explores how Beltane, The Great Rite, and Pagan traditions and laws relate to love and romance. She demonstrates how magical rituals, such as power circles, can help one build self-esteem, attract a fabulous partner, and maintain an exciting relationship of any kind. There are spells and rituals for enhancing sensuality, resolving body image issues, invoking gods and goddesses as sensual consultants, finding balance in relationships, and letting go of old flames. Also included are rituals for boosting fertility and increasing chances of conception, even for those undergoing medical procedures, such as In Vitro Fertilization.

0-7387-0844-5, 288 pp., 6 x 9 $14.95

· ·

To order, call 1-877-NEW-WRLD

Prices subject to change without notice

Charms, Spells & Formulas
For the Making and Use of Gris-Gris Bags, Herb Candles, Doll Magick, Incenses, Oils and Powders
Ray Malbrough

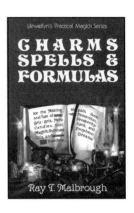

Hoodoo magick is a blend of European techniques and the magick brought to the New World by slaves from Africa. Now you can learn the methods which have been used successfully by Hoodoo practitioners for nearly 200 years.

By using the simple materials available in nature, you can bring about the necessary changes to greatly benefit your life and that of your friends. You are given detailed instructions for making and using the "gris-gris" (charm) bags only casually or mysteriously mentioned by other writers. Malbrough not only shows how to make gris-gris bags for health, money, luck, love, and protection from evil and harm, but he also explains how these charms work. He also takes you into the world of doll magick to gain love, success, or prosperity. Complete instructions are given for making the dolls and setting up the ritual.

978-0-8754-2501-6, 192 pp., 5¼ x 8, illus. $7.95

Also available in Spanish!

. . . .
To order, call 1-877-NEW-WRLD
Prices subject to change without notice

The Beginner's Guide to Sex in the Afterlife
An Exploration of the Extraordinary Potential of Sexual Energy
David Staume

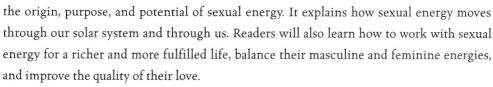

The Beginner's Guide to Sex in the Afterlife is the follow-up to David Staume's quirky and popular *Beginner's Guide for the Recently Deceased.* It assumes, as did his first book, that the reader is dead and takes the reader on a "tour" of the subject.

With humor and intelligence, this guidebook explores the origin, purpose, and potential of sexual energy. It explains how sexual energy moves through our solar system and through us. Readers will also learn how to work with sexual energy for a richer and more fulfilled life, balance their masculine and feminine energies, and improve the quality of their love.

David Staume is a naturopath, herbalist, and writer. He lives in Australia with his family.

978-0-7387-0773-0, 192 pp., 5³⁄₁₆ x 8 $10.95

28 Days to Ecstasy for Couples
Tantra Step by Step
Pala Copeland & Al Link

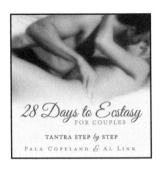

Take your sex life—and your relationship—to new heights in just twenty-eight days! *28 Days to Ecstasy for Couples* can help you and your partner rekindle lost passion, intensify your lovemaking, and experience a sublime spiritual connection.

Perfect for today's busy culture, this step-by-step, illustrated guide to Tantric sex features simple, fun exercises that take twenty minutes or less. Discover how to extend lovemaking, become multiorgasmic, control sexual energy, and engage in sexual, ceremonial, and ritual play. But physical pleasure isn't the only reward. Each activity also includes inspirational messages and lessons in trust, communication, and intimacy.

By practicing sacred love, you'll reap the delights of improved health and vitality and a fulfilling sexual and spiritual relationship.

978-0-7387-0999-4, 192 pp., 7½ x 7½, illus. $17.95

. . . .

To order, call 1-877-NEW-WRLD

Prices subject to change without notice

Sensual Love Secrets for Couples
The Four Freedoms of
Body, Mind, Heart & Soul
Al Link & Pala Copeland

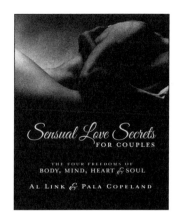

Is it possible to stir up passion after the flames of romantic love die down? How can one maintain a loving relationship that satisfies and stimulates year after year?

Sensual Love Secrets for Couples offers one simple solution for stoking the fires of lifelong intimacy: awakening and uniting the Body, Mind, Heart, and Soul. These four freedoms—the essence of human nature—have the power to transform a lusterless partnership into a divine union sparkling with limitless pleasure and unconditional love. Featuring over one hundred exercises and fun activities, this practical guide helps readers explore the physical senses, establish trust, cultivate emotional intimacy, achieve sacred sex, embrace commitment, pledge selfless intentions, and build spiritual bonds to last a lifetime.

978-0-7387-0965-9, 216 pp., 7½ x 9⅛ $14.95

· ·

To order, call 1-877-NEW-WRLD
Prices subject to change without notice

Hoodoo Mysteries
Folk Magic, Mysticism & Rituals
Ray Malbrough

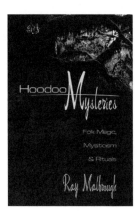

An insider reveals the secrets of Hoodoo. Ray Malbrough, author of the best selling *Charms, Spells, and Formulas*, is one of the few hereditary folk magicians raised in Louisiana. In his latest book, he presents a living history of the magico-religious practices of Louisiana Hoodoo, the American cousin of traditional Haitian Voudoo.

Learn how this religious belief survived as it developed within American shores. Explore the different types of divinatory and magical practices still in use today, including spiritual/magical baths, spellwork for individuals and root doctors, the ritual use of the Pot de Tête (Head Pot) and Medium's Necklace, and invocation of the Gédé (spirits of the dead).

978-0-7387-0350-3, 216 pp., 6 x 9 $14.95

Sticks, Stones, Roots & Bones
Hoodoo, Mojo & Conjuring with Herbs
Stephanie Rose Bird

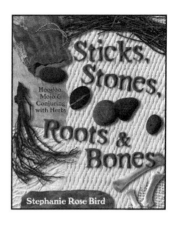

Learn the art of everyday rootwork in the twenty-first century. Hoodoo is an eclectic blend of African traditions, Native American herbalism, Judeo-Christian ritual, and magical healing. Tracing Hoodoo's magical roots back to West Africa, Stephanie Rose Bird provides a fascinating history of this nature-based healing tradition and gives practical advice for applying Hoodoo magic to everyday life. Learn how sticks, stones, roots, and bones—the basic ingredients in a Hoodoo mojo bag—can be used to bless the home, find a mate, invoke wealth, offer protection, and improve your health and happiness.

978-0-7387-0275-9, 288 pp., 7½ x 9⅛, illus. $16.95

To Write to the Author

If you wish to contact the author or would like more information about this book, please write to the author in care of Llewellyn Worldwide and we will forward your request. Both the author and publisher appreciate hearing from you and learning of your enjoyment of this book and how it has helped you. Llewellyn Worldwide cannot guarantee that every letter written to the author can be answered, but all will be forwarded. Please write to:

Kathleen Charlotte
℅ Llewellyn Worldwide
2143 Wooddale Drive, Dept. 978-0-7387-1200-0
Woodbury, MN 55125-2989
Please enclose a self-addressed stamped envelope for reply,
or $1.00 to cover costs. If outside U.S.A., enclose
international postal reply coupon.

Many of Llewellyn's authors have websites with additional information and resources. For more information, please visit our website:

HTTP://WWW.LLEWELLYN.COM

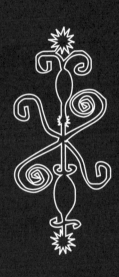